*Psychotherapy with Adolescent Girls
and Young Women*

Psychotherapy with Adolescent Girls and Young Women

Fostering Autonomy through Attachment

Elizabeth Perl

THE GUILFORD PRESS
New York   London

© 2008 The Guilford Press
A Division of Guilford Publications, Inc.
72 Spring Street, New York, NY 10012
www.guilford.com

Printed in the United States of America

This book is printed on acid-free paper.

Last digit is print number: 9 8 7 6 5 4 3 2 1

Library of Congress Cataloging-in-Publication Data

Perl, Elizabeth.
  Psychotherapy with adolescent girls and young women : fostering
autonomy through attachment / Elizabeth Perl.
     p. ; cm.
  Includes bibliographical references and index.
  ISBN-10: 1-59385-651-2 (hardcover : alk. paper)
  ISBN-13: 978-1-59385-651-9 (hardcover : alk. paper)
  1. Adolescent psychotherapy. 2. Teenage girls—Mental health.
  3. Attachment behavior. I. Title.
  [DNLM: 1. Adolescent. 2. Psychotherapy—methods.
  3. Parent–Child Relations. WS 463 P451p 2008]
RJ503.P47 2008
616.89′140835—dc22

                                                              2007047335

About the Author

Elizabeth Perl, PhD, is a board-certified clinical psychologist and an Assistant Professor at Northwestern University's Feinberg School of Medicine. For the past 25 years, Dr. Perl has conducted individual and group psychotherapy in private practice, partial hospital, inpatient, university, and hospital clinic settings. This diverse population has included many adolescent and young adult women with a wide variety of emotional, familial, and relationship problems. Dr. Perl has spoken nationally, published articles, and appeared on television and radio addressing concerns of therapists, graduate students, parents, and young women. She maintains a private practice in Chicago.

Acknowledgments

I have been fortunate to receive support and input from people with very different kinds of connections to adolescent experience: teenage girls who have shared in therapy their current struggles, young women who have shown me that these issues may remain unresolved even in well-functioning adults, mothers in my practice who work to stay connected to daughters while supporting their independent lives, and graduate students who bring perspective from their own adolescent experience and who ask probing and challenging questions as they begin to explore their identities as therapists.

This book grew out of interaction with patients and was shaped by conversation with close colleagues. Shawn Taylor, my longtime group cotherapist and collaborating colleague, knows my clinical work directly and so intimately that she was able to offer her own perspective on my interaction with patients. She brought to this conversation a broad grasp of the literature and a deep understanding of the therapeutic process that clarified or expanded my thinking, and at times even helped me to put into words my own motives for particular spontaneous responses. She also reviewed large parts of the text with painstaking care and attention to detail. Douglas Godfrey generously shared his writing expertise, providing me with invaluable critique and guidance that helped me to more clearly and effectively describe my clinical work. Irwin Hoffman heightened my awareness of more subtle or conflicting underlying influences on a patient and on clinical interaction, challenging me to hold on to multiple perspectives and possibilities so as to better capture the nuanced complexity and ambiguity of therapeutic experience. I also very much appreciate the thoughtful comments and feedback I received from Jean O'Mahoney, Joe Behen, and Peter Zeldow, each of whom reviewed chapters of the book.

Wayne Miller contributed to this work far beyond the role of a supportive spouse. I developed my thinking in endless conversation with him. He always pushed me to be honest about my reactions to patients and to write in a manner that would be understandable to a reader inside or outside of psychology.

Contents

Introduction

Thirteen-year-old Ashley told me that she was tired. She stretched out in her chair, closed her eyes, and fell asleep. So began her seventh weekly psychotherapy session. I expected her to sit up any moment and begin talking, but she did not. As she continued sleeping, I became uncomfortable, even ashamed of what was going on in my office. I imagined her mother's reaction—"This is some expensive nap!" How could I justify the value of such a session? How long should I sit there silently? Perhaps I should wake her and try to explore what she was feeling. Her father had told me that she had argued with her mother and brother during the week. Maybe Ashley did not want to talk about this conflict or her difficulty controlling her temper with her mother.

Yet, as I watched her, I became aware that the experience felt private and strangely intimate. I was free to look at Ashley while she was still, without the distraction of conversation. She seemed softer and more vulnerable. When she sleepily cracked open her eyes, I smiled at her and she smiled back, and then drifted off again. She probably was avoiding some therapeutic work, but she was also creating a haven where she could rest. Had I treated this interaction as resistance, I might have disrupted an opportunity for deepened connection. Ashley drew me into a therapeutic process that I would have been unable to conceive on my own and was initially inclined to resist. We were cuddling without touching. When she returned the next week, she began talking about conflict with her mother and her fear that she could be aggressive when angry. She yawned as she spoke and confirmed that the subject made her tired.

By napping through her session, Ashley was resisting my agenda, which would at least involve some talking. But she might have known better than I did what she needed at that moment. She was looking to me to give her something by remaining engaged as she took the lead. My experience with Ashley illustrates the way that connection with adolescents must be shaped around their own approach to the therapeutic relationship. The therapist participates not primarily by directing the interaction, but by allowing it to happen. The type of bond that is created may not center so much on the therapist's ability to meet particular emotional needs, but on providing a relationship in which each person is seen and accepted. Respect for autonomy is integral to such growth-promoting attachment.

Resistance can represent an expression of self as separate and different from the therapist. I explore the adaptive edge, which can characterize an adolescent's opposition to treatment. A therapeutic breakthrough may be more likely to come from a therapist's effort to engage with and participate in the patient's resistance (e.g., enjoy Ashley's nap) than from any effort to get the patient to relinquish her defensive stance in the moment. When a patient erects a barrier, I not only respect it, but further, I support her efforts to push me back. Although I have never been inclined to override a patient's resistance, I used to be more conflicted than I am now about going along with something that does not fit with my notion of what is therapeutic. For example, with Ashley I might have talked about her napping or interpreted it, thereby pulling our interaction back into a clinical framework that might have been more familiar and comfortable for me. However, I have come to realize that such "therapeutic work" might actually detract from the experience of being present with the patient. When an adolescent is free to be who she is and approach therapy on her own terms, the treatment relationship may be grounded in the experience of therapist and patient as separate but connected.

Before I came to recognize the central role of attachment in facilitating change, I would have regarded Ashley's nap more as a diversion or digression, which I might have tolerated as a means of increasing her sense of control, but would not have valued as a development in our relationship and in the treatment. In fact, I might even have been concerned that by allowing the napping, I was compromising the therapy. Although I now may still hesitate when clinical interaction takes an unanticipated turn, increasingly I recognize that by staying emotionally engaged and receptive, I can offer the patient a vital connection as she works to explore who she is, what she wants from another person, and how to be herself in the context of an intimate relationship. Rather than thinking about her stance merely as resistance, I try to identify expectations I bring to the clinical interaction that could constrain my participation. This reflection hopefully allows me to join with her more fully and discover new experience in our interaction. I am more inclined to forgo my therapeutic agenda to focus on the patient's attachment to me and mine to her.

An adolescent might, for example, be attached to behaviors and relationships that I consider dysfunctional. Although this type of attachment could be understood as resistance, such a perspective emphasizes opposition over adaptive effort. A teenager might need to reject the therapist's perspective and influence in order to assert her autonomy—to be self-directed in the treatment in a way that she has not quite been able to achieve in relation to her mother, perhaps. But there may also be legitimate differences between the viewpoint of the therapist and the patient. As a therapist, I will likely be more attuned to the maladaptive aspects of a behavior or attitude, whereas the patient may be more attuned to adaptive functions including her continuing emotional need to sustain connection to what has been familiar.

The therapeutic relationship may provide an adolescent with her most important attachment outside the family. It can help her move beyond more exclusive emotional dependence on her mother and create a bridge to other nonfamilial attachments. Although I want to be able to influence the adolescent, I have come to realize that it is more important to support her freedom to experience significant control over the development of our relationship—to pace change and to regulate the degree of her dependence and the extent to which she incorporates therapeutic influence. I increasingly have come to recognize the wisdom of the patient's approach to our interaction and to the treatment. She often knows how best to attach and what she needs from me— what feels too close, too overwhelming, too threatening to her autonomy or her sense of loyalty to her mother, and what leaves her feeling too dependent or too vulnerable to regression.

An adolescent girl will bring elements of her struggle with her mother into the treatment relationship. Her willingness to rely on a therapist, to accept therapeutic influence, or to share her feelings will likely be shaped by her relationship with her mother. She may need a caregiving relationship that could provide some of what she has failed to get in her family, reduce her dependence on her mother, or provide a new experience of attachment. It is easy to recognize the patient's attachment needs when she latches on, shows her dependence, and possibly even idealizes the therapist. However, opposition, challenge, and conflict may also reflect her struggle with attachment. Sustained anger or even hostility may allow an adolescent to find a safe outlet for aggression that might otherwise trigger self-destructive behavior and regressive longings.

The teenage girl may therefore reject therapeutic influence, not to defy the treatment, but as a prerequisite or route to attachment. A stance within treatment that defies, creates distance, or limits intimate interaction may help an adolescent tolerate the vulnerability of dependence. Efforts to oppose therapy, therefore, are a defense as well as a part of attachment. In addition, resistance, even defiance, can express autonomy in relation to the therapist, and that is of value in itself. The patient may need the therapist to accept her opposition—not necessarily to agree with her but to respect and engage with her perspective.

If therapists fail to recognize that provocative, oppositional, or rejecting behavior may defend against attachment longings while also expressing effort to develop a sense of self and identity, they may feel that the patient does not need or value them or that they are failing. If they pull back emotionally or propose terminating the treatment, they may deprive the patient of a needed opportunity to reject them while remaining attached. Given an adolescent girl's intense ambivalence about dependence, what appears to be happening in the treatment relationship may be very different from what is actually happening. Anger may mask attachment; self-defeating or destructive behavior may mask an emerging capacity for autonomy. A therapist's protective response, designed to impose some control, might trigger more defiance, thereby increasing the risk of dangerous acting out.

Young Adult or Adult Women May Also Struggle with Disguised Adolescent Issues

Therapists who work with adolescent girls are likely prepared to face unresolved struggles with the mother, ambivalence about attachment and separation, as well as opposition and defiance in the therapy. They expect that longings, frustration, and anger will impact the adolescent's behavior, her sense of herself, and her approach to therapeutic and social relationships. They may not, however, be as attuned to the possible influence of these adolescent struggles on their adult patients. Consequently, therapists may approach the social or professional difficulties experienced by young women as problems of adult adjustment exclusively, rather than as involving possibly disguised unresolved adolescent issues.

These young women may no longer cling to, or fight with, their mothers. In fact, they might be independent, sociable, and successful. There may be no evidence of the provocative, defiant, or self-destructive behavior so characteristic of the period of adolescence. Yet whereas the daughter's struggle with her mother may become tamer and muted as she enters adulthood, it may nonetheless continue to influence her emotional and social functioning. Thus, if therapists fail to recognize unresolved underlying adolescent issues, they may lose a valuable and important opportunity to tackle the root of the patient's problems.

At twenty-nine years of age, Hillary seemed to have successfully navigated the transition to adulthood. She worked as an attorney for city government and was married and planning to have a baby. The marital problems that brought her to treatment seemed to represent a struggle with the challenges of adult life. Despite her reservations about her husband, Tom, and the volatile nature of their fights, she was determined to make her marriage work. This determination could be taken as a sign of her capacity for adult commitment. Yet their relationship was unstable. Their arguments would turn vicious, driving Hillary back to her parents. Subsequent phone conversations would resolve nothing, but she would return to Tom because she was panicked about losing him, thereby ensuring that the cycle of anger, separation, fear of potential loss, and eventual reunion would repeat.

Hillary was unable to use couple therapy to break from this pattern because her marital problems were rooted in deeper issues from her adolescent relationship with her mother. She could not imagine living on her own, so she rushed into marriage as soon as she graduated from college, shifting her emotional and financial dependence from her parents to Tom. By marrying for the purpose of seeking validation and love, she was not developing her ability to meet her needs outside of a caregiving relationship. Elements of dependence on mother will inevitably be carried into adult relationships. But Hillary perpetuated asymmetry in relationships, particularly with men, as the press of her own needs limited her investment in cultivating mutuality.

Hillary believed that her main problem was her marriage, even more specifically, her husband's failure to meet her emotional needs. I believed that she was counting on Tom too exclusively, at the expense of other interests and relationships. She was perpetuating her reliance on a parent-like figure, and this dynamic of reliance retained the asymmetrical structure of her relationship with her mother. Because she felt that she could not live without Tom, she could not stand up for herself in their relationship and set appropriate limits. The therapy, therefore, needed to look beyond her marital problems to confront ways that she brought unresolved childhood longings into adult relationships, which made it difficult for her to tolerate her partner's appropriate needs and limitations in his ability to care for her.

Women may continue to struggle with adolescent issues well into adulthood, even old age. In their twenties and thirties, young women are immersed in the transition to autonomy, as they take on the challenge of finding a romantic partner and a job, achieving financial independence, building a support network outside the family, and taking charge of their emotional and physical health. If they remain too dependent on parental approval or too emotionally tied to family, daughters may be unable to fully embrace committed, intimate peer relationships or pursue their own independent passions. If they are too disconnected or angry with parents, they may lack the secure base that could allow them to take the risks and weather the frustration and disappointment that may be required to succeed with independent ventures.

A young woman who continues to struggle with dependency longings might undermine her own efforts to achieve her goals. Adolescent conflicts may come into play here, as attachment to dysfunctional family relationships or roles may lead to poor romantic or professional choices motivated by unconsciously driven efforts to provoke familiar responses. Difficulties separating from parents can, in this way, cause a young woman to re-create aspects of her family experience, including those that she most wants to escape. If she is ready to change her role in relation to her family and develop her own identity, she may be able to use therapeutic insight to break with familiar patterns and embrace opportunities for new experience.

However, a young woman may become locked in dogged pursuit of a particular adult milestone, such as marriage or having a baby. The goal takes on more importance than the task of developing emotional and social capacities for intimacy, self-reliance, and mutuality. Although the outcome of her efforts may not necessarily be completely within her control, she also may flounder because she is unprepared to take on the emotional challenge of that which she is aiming to achieve. She might be trying to latch on to an external source of purpose, rather than directing her life from within.

Many young women seek help because they have not been able to find a boyfriend who wants to marry them. Marriage may represent an avenue along which a young woman can continue to develop her capacity for mutuality and intimacy. However, if she feels that her life is entirely lacking because she remains single, then marriage might represent something other than what it appears. Lack of success in this arena may leave the young woman feeling that there is something wrong with her. The socially valued path of marriage and family can represent the brass ring for women—evidence that they are loved, valued, and successful, a means to connect with and be like mother, a route to security, and a built-in sense of purpose. Marriage can make a young woman feel both autonomous and cared for, and might seem even more essential when there is a fear of functioning independently or living alone. The desire to find a spouse and create a family may reflect an appropriate adult wish to nurture and be nurtured. But looking to these roles as her sole source of purpose and self-esteem may, in fact, entail avoiding the adolescent task of exploring her own identity and place in the world. If she sees no other route to finding meaning and value in her life, a young woman may become desperate to marry.

Under this pressure, therapists may shrink their perspective to accommodate such a single-minded focus. If therapists fall into the trap of evaluating the therapy based on the patient's ability to achieve this particular goal, they can readily experience the treatment as a failure. They may look at the patient's inability to find a boyfriend as the primary problem, rather than the desperation itself. The patient may be looking to the marital relationship to provide self-esteem and life direction that she should be able to provide for herself.

Therapy can help a young woman expand her thinking, consider different possibilities and directions for her life, and in doing so, further develop her identity. Pursuing a more mutual relationship with a partner might mean that she would need to consider relationships with people she might have ruled out, based exclusively on a wish to be cared for and loved or to impress parents or friends. As she becomes increasingly able to meet these needs autonomously, she may be able to explore a more diverse range of options, free from constraints imposed by the effort to find a replacement for her relationship with her mother or father. Love relationships can then foster genuine mutuality and companionship. She may explore possibilities that are different from her parents and their choices—perhaps a husband who is a peer and friend, a married life without children, a romantic relationship with a woman, a career path she previously could only imagine—independent choices that allow her to choreograph her own life.

Therapists can underestimate the importance of their bond when a young woman is focused on getting her needs met outside of treatment, just as they might with an angry, resistant adolescent who insists that the therapist is not meeting her needs. As a patient expresses despair about what is lacking in her adult life, she may be attaching to the therapist. Although she may need therapeutic help to recognize self-defeating patterns and the potentially undermining influence of dysfunctional family attachments, she may also need the therapist to tolerate her frustration, sadness, and skepticism regarding the therapeutic process. In this way, the therapist can provide a stable base of attachment that is not shaken by the patient's negative reactions. When therapists understand the progressive function of apparently regressive or dysfunctional behaviors, they can then help the patient embrace transitional steps in which repetition can be used to gradually move toward new experience.

Synopsis of the Book

This book is based on my participation, over the last 25 years, in group and individual therapy with adolescent and young adult women in a wide variety of therapeutic settings. The clinical work that I describe is drawn from private practice, partial hospital, inpatient, and university and hospital clinics. Across this demographically, ethnically, and economically diverse population of young women who operate at different levels of functioning with very different kinds of problems, the struggle around attachment and self-direction repeatedly came to the foreground in therapeutic interaction. By providing patients with an experience of connection and separation that differs from that which they had with their mothers, therapists may help young women develop their sense of self (including points of divergence from caregivers), their capacity for mutuality and love outside the family, and their ability to function independently, pursuing professional and creative interests. Throughout the book, I use composite examples to explore these struggles in depth as they unfold in the therapeutic relationship, highlighting pitfalls and opportunities in work with this population.

In the first chapter I describe the intense nature of a daughter's bond with her mother (in contrast to that of a son, who separates from the mother in childhood to attach to, and identify with, the father). The more complex nature of girls' struggles with separation may account for the type of emotional difficulties they experience in adolescence and young adulthood and their resistance to establishing a therapeutic attachment. I explore the ways that dynamics of the mother–daughter relationship may play out in treatment (even with a male therapist). This chapter helps to build an understanding of female adolescent development, specifically the family and emotional influences that support healthy separation and autonomy. It serves as a foundation for the clinically focused description of case examples and therapeutic issues in the rest of the book.

The next three chapters deal with resistance, which can be seen as a daunting obstacle to clinical work, especially with adolescents. To avoid falling into power struggles, therapists must recognize the adaptive functions of resistance. In Chapter 2, I consider therapeutic opposition as a means of asserting autonomy, managing potentially overwhelming feelings of dependence and longings to regress, and preserving longstanding attachments (that may seem dysfunctional to the therapist). By trying to embrace resistance, therapists can build an attachment and support the patient's efforts to control the treatment and to pace change.

Chapter 3 addresses the role of parents in the daughter's resistance, which can be a particular problem when the therapist is working solely with the daughter. The effort to maintain a boundary around the adolescent's treatment so as to protect her privacy and autonomy in relation to the family can limit the therapist's ability to address parental opposition or negative reactions to change—and this limitation can ultimately threaten the viability of the treatment. Therefore, I discuss considerations regarding the parents' involvement in their daughter's therapy.

Chapter 4 shifts the focus from embracing resistance, which at some point begins to limit growth, to challenging resistance as the therapeutic attachment becomes more resilient. As they explore the patient's capacity to let go of dysfunctional attachments, therapists must be prepared to deal with the possibility that they could be threatening the patient's emotional stability and the therapeutic alliance.

As a young woman becomes more attached to her therapist, she may also feel more vulnerable and threatened by growing regressive longings. Chapter 5 explores anger that may be directed toward the therapist, providing a perspective on the function of negative reactions that might help therapists stay emotionally engaged despite the frustration and injury. Even persistent anger may not reflect any problem with the treatment. An adolescent may need to use a therapist as an outlet for anger that would otherwise be directed toward herself in the form of self-destructive behavior. Her anger may also serve to assert autonomy and create distance in the therapeutic relationship reducing the patient's sense of dependence.

However, there is also risk that a patient may attach to a position in therapy that revolves around destructive patterns or persistent threats. In Chapter 6, I explore my effort to determine whether a regressive turn in the treatment relationship has therapeutic value or whether the treatment might be feeding destructive impulses.

Chapter 7 turns to positive expressions of attachment. I consider how the therapist might foster the development from idealization to the experience of more genuine intimacy and mutuality within a caregiving relationship.

The eighth chapter examines the problem of repetition as a young woman works to emerge from the constraints of familiar patterns in therapy and in relationships she creates outside her family. I describe the way in which new experience can emerge from repetition, creating potential for change even in the midst of dysfunctional interaction within therapeutic or social relationships.

After working to establish and deepen their attachment, patients eventually leave the therapist. Termination can repeat elements of the adolescent's struggle to separate from the mother, creating an opportunity for new experience to use attachment to support autonomy. In Chapter 9, I discuss the importance of maintaining a connection in the face of separation, accepting the limits of what therapy can provide, and embracing the patient's responsibility to continue to find ways to grow on her own.

Chapter 1

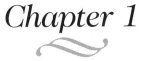

The Mother–Daughter Bond and Its Implications for Understanding the Therapeutic Relationship

With even the smallest provocation, Emily could become wildly angry with her mother. She resented her mother's guidance and rejected her help, yet, even at twenty-one years of age, it was not clear that she could survive on her own. Emily fought parental control by failing to care for herself. This type of rebellion was particularly dangerous because she suffered from juvenile diabetes. Her determination to flaunt dietary restrictions and abuse alcohol endangered her health. Emily's defiance did not liberate her. In fact, she was making it difficult for her parents to shed their sense of responsibility for her. Her parents recognized that their protective efforts could fuel more rebellion, yet they could not trust her to manage independently. Emily fought dependence, but she also refused to assume adult responsibilities.

Emily's struggle to separate from her mother was particularly

intense. Her diabetes had heightened and prolonged her dependence. When she was fifteen, she received a transplant from her
mother, in which part of her mother's organ was used to replace
her own liver. Her mother had made a huge sacrifice for her, and
it was possible that Emily's anger defended against feelings of
guilt and indebtedness. She recovered physically but became sullen, depressed, and antagonistic toward her mother.

The dilemma facing her parents was extreme, as were the
risks associated with Emily's conflicted attempts to assert her
independence. However, in adolescence, all young women face
the struggle that fueled Emily's destructive behavior. They may
make risky and self-defeating choices as they ambivalently pursue
an independent path. To defend against dependent longings, the
teenager may try to detach, rejecting needed help and support—
which may compromise her ability to establish independent functioning.

A close bond with the mother makes the struggle for autonomy more complex and conflicted. Because girls tend to be more
identified with, and attached to, their mothers than are boys, they
will have more difficulty with this adolescent transition. The
struggle to establish an independent identity can persist into
adulthood, particularly when the attachment to the mother has
been conflicted or insecure. It may be expressed differently in
young adulthood than in adolescence, but the underlying conflicts may be similar.

A young woman may flounder with aspects of her social,
romantic, or professional life not because she is ill-equipped to
handle these challenges, but because she is conflicted about establishing an independent identity or forming attachments outside
the family. Rather than trying to create distance in her relationship with her mother by directly challenging established patterns
and expectations, she may make self-defeating choices that contribute to personal or professional frustration or failure. From this
perspective, her difficulty navigating the transition to adulthood
may represent a defensive effort to remain loyal and primarily
attached to her mother.

The adolescent, by contrast, may act out her conflict about
separating through fights with her mother and open defiance. Her
upheaval may be more visibly apparent in her relationship with
her mother, more provocative and dramatic. Girls may direct their

acting out toward their bodies and engage in behaviors that are outside of the domain of parental control. They are at increased risk for eating disorders, reckless or promiscuous sexual activity, and self-cutting or other forms of mutilation. Adolescents may also use drugs and alcohol to rebel, explore, and escape painful feelings. Self-defeating or destructive behavior may provide an illusion of independence while also serving to defend against regressive longings. The thrill and power of reckless acting out can reduce their sense of vulnerability and distract from feelings of loss associated with the transition from childhood dependence.

As they try to deal with these behaviors, mothers can be caught in a conflict between trying to protect and trying to let go. When parents attempt to reassert control, they can inadvertently gratify the adolescent's regressive, dependent wishes. Self-destructive rebellion can protest parental efforts to intervene while provoking more intervention. As the escalating risk triggers more aggressive, protective measures, these measures trigger more defiance and parent and child can become trapped in a vicious cycle.

Therapists working with young women can become caught in a bind that is similar to that of the mother. The attachment to a therapist can take pressure off the mother–daughter dyad, as some dependence needs are being met in a relationship outside the family. However, the stage is then set for the adolescent to re-create with the therapist elements of her struggle with her mother. Her dependence on the therapist can trigger resistance to treatment. Like the defiance at home, acting out within therapy may serve both to rebel against therapeutic influence and to pull for protective intervention.

Although a therapeutic bond will be less longstanding and intense than the mother–daughter bond, therapists are nonetheless subject to strong, conflicting emotional reactions. Therapists are impacted by patients' acting out, by their efforts to reject therapeutic input, and by the risks that patients assume. Like parents, therapists may struggle to support adolescents' autonomy while maintaining an attachment.

After a few months of treatment, Emily began to direct toward me a toned-down version of the rebellion she directed toward her mother. She would report worrisome symptoms of depression and then fail to show for her session. I would call her.

If she answered, we might try to conduct the session over the phone, which made our connection feel even more tenuous. I was trying to stay engaged with her, but in the process, I was also taking too much responsibility for the therapy. She would assure me that she would make her next appointment, only to fail again. I could not maintain the kind of consistent contact or sense of trust needed to build a therapeutic alliance. Like her mother, I felt helpless, frustrated, angry, and concerned.

I became increasingly doubtful that Emily would be able to attach to me and use therapy to establish independence. Her difficulties with self-care hampered her ability to engage in treatment—she could not mobilize to make appointments. I recognized that she might require a more comprehensive intervention, such as a partial hospital that might provide interdisciplinary team treatment in a structured, full-day program of group and individual psychotherapy (with some focus on coping and independent living skills). Multiple therapeutic caregivers might provide an opportunity for attachment that was less concentrated in any one person, such as her mother or me. Emily might be able to resist regressive longings if she were able to turn to a number of professional caregivers (instead of her mother) throughout the day. But I also suspected that she would reject this plan for more comprehensive care. She had refused even lower levels of help and steps that could free her from her dependence on her mother.

Emily posed extraordinary difficulties in therapy. Yet, her underlying struggle is characteristic of adolescents facing the transition to adulthood. A young woman may need a therapist to help her separate from her mother. By providing an additional attachment, therapists can moderate a daughter's dependence. Like a father, they can buffer the attachment to and conflict with mother (Abelin, 1971; Perl, 1998). Therefore, therapists' ability to form and sustain an attachment in the face of resistance is of paramount importance. Yet, they cannot escape the risk that therapeutic attachment could also trigger regression.

The adolescent's tendency to re-create the mother–daughter struggle around attachment and autonomy with a therapist presents both an opportunity and a risk for treatment. The pitfalls of the adolescent's relationship with her mother can, and probably will, repeat. But there is also potential to achieve better resolution of conflict around dependence with the mother, which can reduce the strain on family relationships. The young woman's press toward autonomy may then be guided by healthy mother–daughter attachment rather than an ill-fated attempt to deny or take flight from this bond.

This book explores the particular challenges of therapeutic work with adolescent girls and young women who tend to resist attachment even as they fear independence and separation. I describe my efforts to negotiate a balance between inviting connection and respecting the patient's need to limit dependence and assert her autonomy. Throughout the book, I draw on clinical examples to illustrate the pitfalls and dilemmas therapists will likely encounter as they try to create an attachment and deal with the particular struggles that adolescents introduce into treatment. The following questions target some of the therapeutic problems that I address in subsequent chapters:

- How might a therapist approach attachment with a young woman who is caught in her bond with her mother, governed by family loyalty, and driven to resist any additional dependent tie?
- As therapists foster attachment, they may face intense ambivalence. While resenting her dependence, the patient may long to regress, looking to the therapist to rescue her. How might a therapist understand and deal with the anger, longing, resentment, and resistance stimulated by therapeutic attachment?
- As therapists cultivate dependence and attachment, how can they support autonomy, maximizing the patient's capacity for independent functioning and preparing her to eventually end treatment?

This first chapter serves as a base for understanding female development in adolescence and young adulthood, particularly the nature of the struggle to separate from mother and establish an independent identity. This discussion provides a launching point for the exploration of clinical examples in the chapters to follow. In this first chapter, I identify the challenges that will face therapists who are dealing with this population. In the chapters to follow, I describe how to work through these problems in therapy.

The Mother–Daughter Relationship
Is Re-created in Therapy

The mother–daughter relationship in adolescence provides a basis for understanding the therapeutic relationship. Regardless of the therapist's gender, aspects of the mother–daughter relationship are likely to be re-created in therapy. The most critical factor in the development of a treatment relationship is therapist's capacity for attachment. The opportunity to attach to an adult outside the family can impact the patient's relationship with her mother. A male is no less able than a female to provide an alternative attachment, and some version of the problems from her relationship with her mother will be inclined to repeat in any close treatment relationship.

Mothers must deal with the vulnerability of sustaining attachment in the face of impending separation. Therapists must try to build an attachment with an adolescent who is intent on protecting and asserting her emerging sense of autonomy. A mother's past experience with attachment and the emotional needs and vulnerabilities that she brings to her relationship with her daughter will influence the kind of attachment she offers, which in turn will influence the daughter's approach to relationships. Slade (1999) acknowledges that attachment dynamics also influence a therapist's feelings about and response to the patient. She explains that therapists bring their own vulnerabilities and attachment histories to the treatment relationship (p. 586), which similarly shape the quality of their attachment to the adolescent.

As familiar patterns are reenacted within the treatment relationship, a paradigm of normal female adolescent development can provide a valuable reference point. The patient may resist therapeutic attachment in much the same way that she fights her tie with her mother. Although offering a haven separate from the mother, the treatment relationship is similarly fraught with risk of regression and repetition. A young woman may desperately need an attachment with an alternative caregiver, but she may fear depending on a therapist.

There is no one optimal way for an adolescent to utilize a therapeutic relationship. Like the parent, a therapist cannot be sure of the patient's needs or motives at any particular juncture. An intense therapeutic connection could reflect a successful attachment that will be used eventually to launch social relationships, or it could represent a retreat from social opportunities. A patient could experience a therapeutic intervention as an attempt to undermine rather than support her autonomy. Moreover, it may be difficult to determine whether defiance is progressive or regressive.

A young woman may try to minimize her vulnerability by disguising her attachment. She may appear to be indifferent to therapeutic influence when, in fact, she cares very much what the therapist thinks about her. When an adolescent spends an entire session talking about her friends without seeking any input from me, for example, I do not assume that she is uninterested in my thoughts and reactions. In fact, she may be so concerned that she tries to preclude feedback. A critical reaction could be too injurious, and she may value an enthusiastic response so much that she could feel pressured to sustain it. She may need to talk so intently about her friends in the first place because she is trying to manage feelings of dependence on me. Or she may want to share her social life because she feels close. When an adolescent cancels a session to engage in some activity, I might not confront her decision as resistance or explore its meaning in terms of her feelings about therapy, as I might with an adult. Rather, I would support her interests outside of treatment while also recognizing that she may need to prioritize peers or independent pursuits to be able to sustain our attachment.

If therapists challenge the patient's failure to prioritize treatment, they might re-create the adolescent's experience with a parent who pressured her to subordinate independent interests to family involvement. By supporting the adolescent's decisions regarding her treatment, therapists can support her autonomy. To this end, therapists must be willing to take a back seat to the patient's other commitments without reducing their investment or availability. When an adolescent is free to push away from the therapist without compromising the treatment relationship, she may experience a more secure sense of attachment.

The Need for Ongoing Attachment to a Caregiver

We used to believe that adolescents must relinquish ties to parents to create love relationships with peers and take their place in the adult world. Anna Freud (1975) suggested that healthy development demands "gradual detachment" that leaves adolescents with "a passionate longing for partnership which they succeed in transferring to the environment outside the family" (p. 134). Blos (1968) conceptualized the need to "disengage from infantile object ties" as part of "the second individuation process of adolescence" (p. 252). By drawing on Mahler's concept of "separation–individuation" in the first years of life, Blos was emphasizing the similarities between the struggle of the teenager and that of the young child to move toward age-appropriate separation from the mother. These traditional psychoanalytic theories have emphasized the need for adolescents to *detach*—to give up their childhood dependence and rely instead on what they have internalized.

More contemporary theorists have challenged this viewpoint. Marohn (1998) suggests that adolescents relate to parents differently as they approach adulthood—while remaining attached. "Traditional theory tells us that adolescents should separate and individuate—that they should 'give up' childhood claims and 'grow up.' Yet somehow patients, friends, children, and research subjects don't behave that way" (p. 15). Childhood attachments need not be sacrificed in the service of establishing independence.

The press to relinquish such connections might heighten feelings of insecurity and vulnerability, undermining the adolescent's capacity to maintain stable autonomy. Marohn (1998) explains that teenagers become uneasy when they believe that they "should be 'breaking' their ties to their parents—and they are not disposed to do so" (p. 15). The caregiving bond, from this perspective, is never outgrown but, rather, becomes the basis for adult attachments. The young adult "has not psychologically separated from her mother and become an autonomous individual with no further tie to mother; rather, she has built on that tie, modified that bond, and calls on it regularly to serve as a template from which to forge and shape new relationships while preserving aspects of the old" (Marohn, 1998, p. 12).

Benjamin (1988) also challenges the traditional psychoanalytic theory that adolescents will progress from attachment to detachment—a theory that emphasizes autonomy at the expense of relatedness. "It implies an autonomous individual defined by [her] ability to do without the 'need-satisfying object.' The other seems more and more like a cocoon or a husk that must gradually be shed—one has got what one needs, and now, goodbye" (p. 43). Benjamin suggests that autonomy develops not in the absence of connection but rather in the context of ongoing relationship. Paradoxically, perhaps, adolescents look to their parents to recognize and validate their independence. Parental capacity to appreciate the daughter as a separate person can enrich the quality of their attachment.

Parents' continuing importance may not be as evident as daughters begin to turn to peers. The adolescent may confide less in parents and spend less time with them relative to friends, but her social development may nonetheless depend on this ongoing familial connection. A secure attachment allows the adolescent to relegate her relationship with parents to the background and draw on their support as needed. In this way, she may rely not only on an internalized sense of connection to parents but on an ongoing attachment, as well. If she feels loved by her parents, she will be more able to love others and to feel loved by her peers.

Parents as a Secure Base for Exploration

The connection between attachment and autonomy becomes evident in the first years of life, and our understanding of adolescence in this regard is grounded in the study of the mother–child relationship. Ainsworth (1963) first described the infant's use of an attachment figure as a "secure base" from which to explore. This pioneering research described the way in which an infant uses the mother as a base "from which to explore the environment during times of safety and from which to seek comfort and security at times of stress" (Lyons-Ruth, 1991, p. 4). Bowlby (1988) recognized the importance of the physical presence of the mother and also, at times of separation, the child's belief that the mother will be available if needed. The need for this sense of connection persists even as we become independent. "This concept of the secure personal base, from which a child, an adolescent, or an adult goes out to explore and to which [she] returns from time to time, is one that I have come to regard as crucial for an understanding of how an emotionally stable person develops and functions *all through [her] life*" (Bowlby, 1988, p. 46; italics in original).

Mahler (1979) believed that the infant is "hatched" from mother's "symbiotic orbit" and must struggle to individuate and develop a separate sense of self (p. 86). She described the role of the mother as providing a "stable point" or "home base" (p. 124). Mahler's concept of "refueling" (p. 124) is based on recognition of a continuing need for access to caregiving in the service of developing independence. For a child to fully exercise her autonomous capacities, she must know that the parent is available as needed.

Lyons-Ruth (1991), a more contemporary infant researcher, suggested that Mahler's separation–individuation model of development might be better conceptualized as a process of "attachment–individuation." Lyons-Ruth explains that this terminology "emphasizes the infant propensity to establish and preserve emotional ties to preferred caregivers at all costs, while simultaneously attempting to find a place within these relationships for his or her own goals and initiatives" (p. 8). This perspective implies a more emotionally driven hunger for connection to the mother, beyond the need to refuel.

Building on the work of Lyons-Ruth, Doctors (2000) asserted that "the sense of connection and sense of distinctiveness develop in tandem" (p. 5). She explains that "security of attachment promotes firmer individuation and vice versa" (p. 11). Attachment and individuation are therefore "mutually strengthening" (p. 13).

Benjamin (1988) affirmed the continuing need for parental connection, emphasizing the role of more nuanced, emotional aspects of the parent–child relationship, particularly the mother's ability to attune to the emotional experience of the child as the child explores the world.

> The baby who looks back as [she] crawls off toward the toys in the corner is not merely refueling or checking to see that mother is still there, but is wondering whether the mother is *sharing* the feeling of [her] adventure—the fear, the excitement, or that ambiguous "scarey-wonderful" feeling. The sense of shared feeling about the undertaking is not only a reassurance, but is, itself, a source of pleasurable connection. (Benjamin, 1988, p. 31; italics in original)

These same questions pertain to the parent's role in supporting the development of autonomy in adolescence. Mahron's recognition of the importance of continuing connection for adolescents would fit with Lyons-Ruth's concept of attachment–individuation. Teenagers need their parents for refueling, but their sense of self and capacity for relationships are also tied to ongoing connection. The exploration that takes place in adolescence is in large part social, and the bond with parents provides the foundation of love and acceptance that may allow teenagers to invest emotionally in their peers. Secure attachment to parents supports a daughter's ability to tolerate the stress and volatility of social interaction. If a teenager were to expose her needy feelings and regressive longings to peers, she would risk rejection or ridicule. But if she can turn to parents with these more childlike emotional needs, seeking regressive gratification in this secure haven, she will be able to relate to peers in a manner that will more likely assure her acceptance.

Leah, a popular seventeen-year-old girl, confided to me that she could not manage her social life if she did not know that her parents were behind her. She explained that she loves her friends but that they "go up and down" emotionally. Leah accepts their moodiness and even enjoys the "drama," but she recognizes that the relationships are unstable. In school, Leah was rarely the target of anger or critical judgment, but she was nonetheless unsettled by the shifting alliances, betrayals, and backbiting among her friends. She was a loyal friend and she believed that her girlfriends would be there for her, to look out for her if she gets drunk or to "hang out" with her, but she also acknowledged that teenagers are selfish. Leah admitted that she complains about her parents and she fights with them, but she also knows that they will always support her, even when they are angry. She acknowledged that she cannot count on her friends in that way.

Attachment Problems within the Family Complicate a Daughter's Efforts to Launch

When parents remain emotionally engaged and attached even in the face of adolescent rebellion, they create opportunity for their daughter to more securely push for autonomy. By detaching, parents might appropriate initiative for separation, thereby

disempowering the adolescent—a daughter cannot push away
from parents who have disengaged from her. The emotional vulnerability that may motivate a parent's need to detach can also
inhibit a daughter's independent initiative. A teenager may be
wary of asserting her autonomy if she believes that her defiance or
efforts to individuate might hurt her parents or be experienced as
abandonment. Ryan and Lynch (1989) emphasize the role of emotional connection for adolescent development. "Some forms of
detachment from the family are associated with an experienced
lack of parental support and acceptance, which not only does not
conduce to independence and autonomy but may actually interfere with the consolidation of identity and the formation of a positive self-concept" (p. 340).

Yet, it is understandable that parents might be inclined to
detach when an adolescent begins to challenge their authority or
resist their influence. By disengaging from the rebellious teenager,
parents protect themselves from the emotional impact of rejection
and the loss of idealization. They may defensively adopt a more
indifferent or laissez faire stance, which may help them tolerate
the defiance. However, the adolescent is then deprived of the
opportunity to tangle with the parent and to bring autonomy into
their relationship. "The parent who cannot tolerate the child's
attempt to do things independently will make the child feel that
the price of freedom is aloneness, or even, that freedom is not
possible" (Benjamin, 1988, p. 36). Injured parents may withdraw
because they believe that their child no longer needs them. Faced
with such parental vulnerability, a daughter may believe that she
must sacrifice her independence to stay connected to parents.

When the adolescent does not feel securely attached to parents, she may seek support and acceptance outside the family,
attempting to create a family among her peers. She may turn to
older teens or young adults who are also seeking to compensate
for deficits in their family connections. Although the effort to
form sustaining relationships is adaptive, premature reliance on
peers poses risks. Even if they are older and trustworthy, peers
will lack the stability and nurturing focus of a parent. Yet, friendships may become primary because they may constitute the best
support available.

Rather than disengaging appropriately in a healthy way to
allow for growing independence, some parents react to the adoles-

cent's budding autonomy by trying to hold onto control and centrality in her life. When parents are unable to tolerate the loss of their role as a primary source of comfort or nurturing, they may retain control via overgratification. Benjamin (1988) argues that parental efforts to continue to meet all the needs of their child can undermine not only the development of autonomy but also the daughter's sense of herself as a separate person.

> The self-obliteration of the permissive parent who cannot face this blow does not bring happiness to the child who gets everything [she] demands. The parent has ceased to function as an other who sets a boundary to the child's will . . . the parent co-opts all the child's intention by agreement, pushing [her] back into an illusory oneness where [she] has no agency of [her] own. (Benjamin, 1988, p. 35)

By attempting to gratify the needs of an adolescent, parents communicate that she should remain dependent. The daughter may feel less confident about her ability to meet her own needs or may experience such independence as a threat to her parents. If parents invite continued reliance on their resources and caregiving, they reduce the teenager's motivation to tolerate the inevitable deprivation, frustration, and stress experienced in efforts to meet her own needs. Parents need to temper the comfort and gratification they provide with a willingness to step back and allow the adolescent to struggle. They should aim to provide "optimal autonomy in the context of emotional support" (Ryan & Lynch, 1989, p. 341), allowing the adolescent to assume as much responsibility for her life as she can manage.

The development of such independence within a caregiving relationship allows for more genuine mutuality. Holmes (1996) describes the "reciprocal" relationship between autonomy and intimacy:

> Autonomy is possible on the basis of a secure inner world—we can go out on a limb, stand our ground, make our own choices, and tolerate aloneness if we can be sure that attachment and intimacy are available when needed. Conversely, intimacy is possible if the loved one can be allowed to be separate; we can allow ourselves to get close if we feel autonomous enough not to fear engulfment or attack, and also know that separation does not mean that our loved one will be lost forever. (p. 19)

As she discovers her own capacities and recognizes that she is able to do for herself much of what her parents have done for her, the teenager may begin to deidealize them. The loss of a belief in parental omnipotence can be unsettling but also liberating. When a young woman sees her parents as infallible and herself as fallible, she will feel that she must continue to rely on them. The recognition of parental fallibility makes dependence feel a bit less secure, but it also makes independence seem more possible.

A Hostile–Dependent Bond

Adolescent girls may fluctuate between more adult levels of independence and childlike dependence, making it difficult for parents (or a therapist) to know what they need. Even when parents want to incorporate increasing levels of autonomy into their relationship with their daughter, they cannot always be sure when to hold on and when to let go, when to direct and when to encourage independent decision making, when to set limits and when to trust the adolescent's capacity for self-regulation. Although the adolescent may sometimes be able to communicate what she needs, it is also possible that she will push away when she most needs nurturing or that she will cling at times when she needs to manage more autonomously. Parents may undermine their daughter's independence either by holding on when the adolescent should be exploring, or by being unavailable at a vulnerable juncture.

Moreover, parents can neither predict nor control whether their daughter will accept their support. A daughter may direct her frustration toward her parents, blaming them for her failures and angrily refusing help while also refusing to care for herself. She may have legitimate reason to be angry with her parents. But even if it is reasonable, blame can be used to avoid taking responsibility for her life. Angry, help-rejecting behavior may prolong dependence.

It can be difficult for parents to allow the adolescent to be responsible for the consequences of reckless or negligent choices. Fear and guilt can draw them into a codependent position in which they try to convince the daughter to accept their care. Parents may also have difficulty letting go of longstanding hopes and expectations for their daughter and accepting her limitations. They may become directive in an attempt to get her to achieve beyond her capacity or to follow the path they want for her. If parents cannot accept their daughter's limitations and inclinations, they may compromise her ability to sustain her best level of functioning.

Emily's diabetes and liver transplant made it more difficult for her parents to abdicate their caregiving role. Yet, their protective efforts seemed to have little positive, constructive impact. Even with their supervision, Emily failed to follow a diabetic diet: She drank and smoked pot and was sexually active (all of which presented greater risk because of the liver transplant), and she often skipped medical appointments. Despite her obvious failure in self-care, Emily resented her mother's involvement. Emily's parents recognized that they might be contributing to their daughter's prolonged dependence, yet they reasonably feared that she could become seriously ill if they did not step in.

Emily's health problems restricted her freedom to explore and experiment. She took risks because she wanted to do what her friends did, but she was also anxious about her health. Because of her illness, the prospect of independence was more frightening and less exciting. She could not trust her body. Despite her anger at her parents, she admitted that they were her only source of security—they had always known what to do when she was sick. She feared that even if she took care of herself, she might not be okay, which heightened her ambivalence about being on her own.

Emily struggled with the magnitude of her mother's sacrifice. She felt that she could never (and would not want to) live up to this standard. Consequently, she was reluctant to step up to a more mature position in her relationships, which might include assuming some caregiving responsibility. Although for brief moments Emily could listen empathically and offer emotional support to others, she tended to rely so heavily on her friends to meet her own emotional needs that the relationships would inevitably evolve toward a lopsided focus on her. Her friends might have felt burdened by Emily's depression, loneliness, and doubts about her self-worth. Emily expected a lot, and she was frequently not prepared to give back. As a consequence, her needs would frequently overshadow those of her friends.

She relied on a shared experience of anger or depression to

sustain her peer relationships, which made for tenuous connections. If a friend needed too much or provided too little, Emily
would pull back. If a friend became more successful and happier,
Emily would become bitter and resentful. Rather than supporting
her friend's development, she would withdraw and the relationship would disintegrate.

Emily's rebellion seemed less an expression of autonomy than
a misguided expression of her rage about her limitations. Rather
than working toward self-care and self-sufficiency, which she
feared she could not achieve, she derived a sense of control
through self-destructive behavior. She felt most powerful when
she was fighting her parents, on whom she was able to make an
emotional impact. Any adolescent might direct anger and fear
about her life and future toward parents, but Emily was struggling
with extreme rage. Her diabetes had robbed her of her formerly
carefree spirit, had caused her to fall behind academically and
socially, had made her different from her friends, and forced her to
depend too much on her parents. She had lost motivation to be
independent. In this way, Emily's fear and anger tied her to her
parents in an indefinite state of hostile, help-rejecting dependence.

Emily's willingness to expose this struggle in therapy suggested that she might be attaching to me. As she talked about her
relationship with her mother, she expressed her anger verbally—
which could also represent a step from self-destructive acting out.
She was confiding in me, which represented the beginning of a
connection, but she was so angry that she was unable to relax into
a therapeutic attachment (even though she did not seem angry
with me). Our relationship did not yet carry enough weight to
serve as an anchor, outside her family, that she could use to begin
building her own life. Nor did it seem sufficiently strong to absorb
her anger if she began to direct it toward me. I was not yet, therefore, in a position to help Emily separate from her mother.

The Struggle to Emerge
from the Bond with Mother

Both boys and girls establish a primary attachment to their
mother, but in early childhood, as noted, boys separate and begin

to identify with their father. Boys need to make a break with their mothers to develop a sense of masculine identity. Girls, by contrast, do not need to separate from their mothers in childhood. Because they are the same gender, girls not only attach primarily to their mothers, they also identify primarily with them. Therefore, the mother–daughter bond is particularly close, even from infancy. Because the girl can maintain this attachment to her mother uninterrupted throughout childhood, the task of separating in adolescence becomes a more difficult transition.

Chodorow (1978) emphasizes the strength of attachment between mothers and daughters, suggesting that the mutual identification can create a sense of symbiotic connection:

> Because they are the same gender as their daughters and have been girls, mothers of daughters tend not to experience these infant daughters as separate from them in the same way as do mothers of infant sons. In both cases, a mother is likely to experience a sense of oneness and continuity with her infant. However, this sense is stronger, and lasts longer, vis-à-vis daughters. Primary identification and symbiosis with daughters tend to be stronger . . . that is, to be based on experiencing a daughter as an extension or double of the mother herself. (p. 109)

Benjamin (1988) also acknowledges a symbiotic aspect to the connection between mother and daughters, but highlights the fact that it can coexist with recognition of separateness. A mother may simultaneously experience her infant daughter as being the same as or one with her, but also different and separate. The female baby will feel "part of herself" (the mother), "utterly familiar yet utterly new, unknown and other" (p. 14).

Blos (1962) also recognized that girls struggle more in adolescence with their ties to mothers than do boys because of the intense nature of their bond. He believed that the mother–daughter attachment could complicate efforts to establish primary love relationships outside the family, explaining that the girl's "prolonged and painful severance from the mother constitutes the major task of this period" (p. 66). Therapists today may not think in terms of severing ties, but they have probably witnessed the painful ambivalence and often volatile struggle associated with an adolescent girl's effort to assert an independent identity.

Struggles with mutual identification and feelings of symbiotic connection may characterize a healthy mother–daughter relationship, and conflict is a normal part of this struggle. An adolescent girl may rebel because she is intensely attuned to her mother's feelings and vulnerabilities. In fact, the conflict she provokes may reflect her effort to break from an overwhelming sense of connection—she may fight with her mother to gain needed emotional distance.

Given the nature of a daughter's empathic tie to her mother, there is risk that a mother's unresolved emotional longings may tip the balance of the caregiving relationship too much in the direction of parental needs, introducing a sense of obligation or responsibility that can conflict with the daughter's freedom to pursue autonomy. In short, the adolescent may sacrifice her own interests for her mother. To successfully launch from a family that is too much dominated by parental needs, a daughter may be forced to draw a boundary that allows her to prioritize her own needs, even if she fears that she will hurt her mother. Although she may be disadvantaged by the absence of a secure home base, she may nonetheless be better able to find her own niche than if she focused her efforts on preserving established family roles and ties.

Even healthy families are not free from ambivalence and conflict in response to the evolving relationship between parents and adolescents. It is normal for parents to feel some sadness about the loss. The daughter, struggling with her own ambivalence, may want to cut off her emotional investment or contact with parents to avoid the inevitable longing and pain. Her wish for approval is not necessarily pathological, even if it continues to keep her too tied to her parents. In a healthy family, the daughter does not need to detach, but she may want to, so as to counter her own wishes to retain a primary reliance on the security of these bonds.

If she opts to detach rather than to work on asserting autonomy in the context of continuing attachment, the adolescent may forfeit the opportunity to negotiate more nuanced shifts in her relationship with her mother. It can be easier to disengage than to face disappointing her parents and the temptation to continue to turn to them for security and gratification. Yet, it is not possible to escape these struggles by detaching, moving far away, or even cutting off all ties with parents. Unresolved feelings in relation to the mother can continue to impact the daughter's sense of herself and her ability to embrace social and professional opportunities and commitments well into adult life, even after her parents have died.

A healthy bond allows the adolescent to explore and assert ways in which she is different from, and independent of, the mother while remaining attached. Chodorow (1998) recognized the role that continuing attachment plays in the development of identity. She explained that a girl's identity emerges from her experience of self within relationship:

> Separateness from the mother, defining oneself apart from her (and from other women), is not the only or final goal for women's ego strength and autonomy. In the process of differentiation, leading to a genuine autonomy, people maintain contact with those with whom they had their earliest relationships, where this contact is part of who we are. . . . Differentiation is not distinctness and separateness, but a particular way of being connected to others. (p. 389)

Ties therefore need not be relinquished for a young woman to achieve independence. Feminist writers have recognized the developmental advantage of the daughter's uninterrupted connection to the mother. Girls may cultivate a deeper capacity for attachment through this bond, which can enrich their adult relationships. The sense of self develops in the context of relationship, specifically in conjunction with a sense of the other as a separate person with his or her own needs and feelings.

The ability to articulate a sense of self is therefore tied to a capacity for mutuality. A young woman must become aware of her own needs and feelings, but not in a manner that precludes or supersedes empathic awareness of the needs and feelings of the other. She should grow to be mindful of her own needs and those of the other and to assert differences without being "dominated by felt need and one's own exclusive subjectivity" (Chodorow, 1998, p. 386). As the tie to her mother becomes more mutual, a daughter can learn to moderate her own needs by considering the experience of the other.

These are the very relational qualities that could be developed within treatment. Although caregiving aspects of the therapist's role predominate, as they would with a mother, therapy affords an opportunity to cultivate a reciprocal connection, wherein the patient's needs remain central, but not to a point of denying or ignoring the therapist's needs, feelings, and limits. As I explore my experience of attachment with patients, I describe ways in which I have introduced and supported mutuality, with the patient's participation, thereby expanding the treatment relationship and the roles of patient and therapist.

The close nature of the mother–daughter bond can develop capacity for empathy while also inhibiting social exploration. "Since masculinity is defined through separation while femininity is defined through attachment, male gender identity is threatened by intimacy while female gender identity is threatened by separation" (Gilligan, 1993, p. 8). Girls may be less prepared for, or more conflicted about, separation relative to boys, but better prepared to build mutually supportive relationships. Connection rather than separation becomes the base for building autonomy. A goal of treatment would be to help the adolescent expand beyond attachment to her mother so that she might have the security and confidence to embrace other relationships.

The bond with the mother is at the core of a young woman's struggle to develop her sense of self as she enters adulthood. Their connection may be affectionate or angry, and it may stimulate efforts to be close or distant, dependent or nurturing. But regardless of the tenor of the relationship, this bond will continue to dominate the female's emotional life. The connection with the mother will be internalized, and the young woman may find that her efforts to create her own life repeat patterns from her relationship with her mother and her mother's life.

Erin, a young woman in her early twenties, would tell you without hesitation that her mother (Mrs. D) was her best friend, her confidante and her biggest source of support. She had always turned to Mrs. D when she was lonely or distressed, but recently Erin had been depressed, and she felt uncharacteristically disinclined to share this struggle with her mother. She doubted that her mother could help, but she also admitted that her mother had been "getting on her nerves." Although Erin realized that Mrs. D had always tended to be intrusive, she was now more bothered by her mother's definitive opinions and her wish to direct Erin's life. Erin had also begun to feel frustrated with her friends, with whom she'd been close since elementary school. She valued this shared history, but she nonetheless was feeling increasingly frustrated that they could not understand her current life. She did not know whether her friends and her mother really were failing to meet her needs or whether she was simply irritable from her depression. She had been frustrated like this before, but the feelings had always passed. Now, Erin felt she had stagnated. She had not dated for more than six months, she had not made any new friends since college, and her relationship with her mother and her childhood friends no longer seemed able to meet her needs as they had in the past.

Erin knew that she needed help, but worried that her mother would panic if she realized the extent of her depression and would feel hurt that she wanted to confide in a therapist. Erin believed that her problem was depression. I believed that she was clinically depressed, but it seemed possible that her distress was also a function of increasing need to break free of confining ties to her mother and, more generally, to her childhood, in the service of developing an independent identity and life path. Her symptoms were forcing her to seek involvement outside the family that would have otherwise been unthinkable. From this perspective, Erin's decision to enter treatment in the face of her mother's anticipated negative reactions might have been a first step toward increased autonomy.

With a job in advertising, Erin was financially and professionally successful but still emotionally entwined with her mother. She owned her own apartment but stayed in her old neighborhood to be near her parents. Since childhood, she had been concerned with her mother's needs and feelings, and in adolescence, Erin had increasingly taken on a caregiving role. She had no siblings, which heightened her sense of responsibility. Erin would often devote her weekend time to helping with her mother's business as a wedding consultant and arranger. On these visits, she would also manage their bills and finances, as her parents were strapped with debt and she had more of a head for business than they did.

If her father was drinking heavily, Erin would stay overnight in their home. It was more important for her to support and protect her mother than to protect herself from the stress of their explosive marital conflict. Although her mother often provoked these fights, Erin saw her as a victim because her father was stronger, alcoholic, and abusive. On a few occasions, he had hit his wife. By standing by her mother, Erin tried to reciprocate her mother's devotion to her.

Mrs. D had always made sacrifices to give Erin the means to a better life. But her mother's failure to care for herself, her marriage, and her finances burdened her daughter. Mrs. D may have been unconsciously motivated to make dysfunctional choices to keep her daughter involved in her life. However, Erin also enabled her mother's dependence. Mrs. D was free to overextend herself because she knew that Erin would bail her out. Erin liked to be needed, and she derived a sense of purpose from taking care of her mother.

Erin had her own motives for maintaining a primary attachment to her mother. She feared rejection, especially in dating relationships. She chose partners who seemed to be initially intensely attracted to her, but their attention would quickly turn controlling. She would stay in the relationship even when she began to feel disparaged. Her boyfriend's criticism would make her feel insecure, and this made her cling all the more. She was unconsciously attracted to men who could be aggressive, like her father. Then, like her mother, she failed to set self-protective limits that could be enforced by a willingness to leave.

Outside of her intermittent dating experiences, Erin's social life revolved around childhood relationships. These friends provided companionship but not meaningful emotional support— since high school she had developed in ways that they had not. If she were more socially engaged, she would likely have chosen different friends by this point, but she did not pursue intimacy outside of her relationship with her mother. Her mother always insisted that "you can only trust family." Erin's approach to relationships fulfilled this prophecy and reinforced her continued emotional dependence on her mother.

Erin was frustrated that her mother would not consider leaving her father, or at least set limits with him. I pointed out that Erin repeated this pattern when she stayed involved with disrespectful men, and also when she would unfailingly accommodate her mother's requests, regardless of the impact on her own life. In response to this confrontation, Erin began to question her automatic willingness to provide whatever her mother seemed to need.

She was beginning to develop a more complex view of her mother. Erin continued to see her as a victim, but she also began to doubt that her mother was as helpless as she appeared to be. Increasingly, she recognized that her mother was making choices, some of which had had a profoundly negative impact on Erin's life. She continued to help her mother, but rather than jumping into any crisis, she focused on trying to empower her mother to take better care of herself, her finances, and her business.

Months into her treatment, Erin began to refuse some of her mother's requests. In response, Mrs. D became angry and withdrew, trying to pressure Erin to return to her former accommodating role. But with my support, Erin held her ground and trusted that eventually Mrs. D would accept new terms in their relationship. Although she was hurt by her mother's anger, Erin was reassured that the vigor of Mrs. D's resistance reflected strength that she had not previously witnessed and which her mother could choose to use on her own behalf. Erin also began to recognize that her mother did not always act in consideration of Erin's best interests. Consequently, Erin no longer believed that her mother would do anything for her, and she became liberated from a boundless sense of obligation.

Parental Dependence Can Undermine a Daughter's Autonomy

Even healthy parents will inevitably bring self-serving motives to their relationship with an adolescent. A teenage daughter begins to interact with parents in a more adult manner at about the same time that she begins to turn her focus to peers, which may frustrate parents. It is normal and appropriate for parents to look to an adolescent daughter to meet some of their needs. As parents turn to her more over time, they can create an opportunity for increased mutuality. But parents must moderate their emotional reliance on a daughter. The job of the parents is to help their daughter manage the demands and challenges of more mutual relationships with peers—not to transform the caregiving bond into a reciprocal relationship.

"The last major caregiving task of parents becomes supporting their adolescent's capacity to cope with the affect engendered in learning to live independently of parental caregiving" (Allen & Land, 1999, p. 330). This task extends into adulthood, but over time, even while the daughter continues to rely on secure family attachment, parents fade increasingly into the background. The adolescent's growing independence can expand roles and possibilities for interaction within the family, but parental expectations must be tempered by awareness that the daughter may continue to need to think of the parent as a parent.

When parents look to their daughter to feel needed and loved, important or admired, or to derive security from her dependence, they may feel threatened by signs of growing autonomy. Although they may maintain a caregiving role, they may nonetheless be emotionally dependent on their child. The dominating influence of parental needs may create a "role reversal." In the extreme, adults may cling to their children in an attempt to derive security from them (Cassidy & Berlin, 1994, p. 980).

Parents must remain attuned to the adolescent's independent experience and be ready to step in, but in response to their daughter's needs rather than their own. Unresolved parental dependency needs may cause parents to sabotage their daughter's growing independence. A parent who is threatened by the child's emerging autonomy may be systematically unavailable when she is most needed and intrusively present when she is not, thereby reinforcing dependent behavior and subtly discouraging independent behavior. The mother may be oblivious to the daughter's needs. But it is also possible that she may be using her ability to home in on the daughter's emotional experience to undermine the daughter's efforts to separate.

The mother's capacity for emotional attunement, and the way she uses her sensitivity, influences adolescent development much in the way it does in infancy. Observations from mother–infant interaction are therefore applicable to the development of autonomy in adolescence. Cassidy and Berlin (1994) well summarize this point:

> The mother's selective ignoring of her infant's interest in autonomous exploration may reflect the fact that attention to such signals would disrupt a model in which mother–child closeness is of prime importance. . . . If a mother (consciously or unconsciously) wants to be particularly assured of her importance to the infant, of [her] dependency on [the mother], and of [her] availability to meet [mother's] own attachment needs, a high efficient parental strategy is one of low or intermittent responsiveness. . . . A parent with a conscious or unconscious desire to prolong the baby's need for her will not quickly respond to attachment behavior. [The resulting] clinginess may annoy but also fulfill mother's needs and provides comfort. (p. 984)

These dynamics may play out in more nuanced ways as a child develops. Cassidy and Berlin (1994) describe the way in which intangible influences, such as parental insensitivity to cues and subtle seduction, can shape the nature of the adolescent's attachment and her confidence in her own autonomous abilities:

> Beyond infancy, maternal insensitivity may increasingly take the form of ignoring the child's signals for autonomy and overemphasizing the parent–child relationship. The parent of an older child, who may be by this time a dependent, clingy child, may then emphasize the intimacy and specialness of the relationship and become much more (perhaps overly) involved with the child. (p. 984)

A daughter may also be attuned to the impact of her growing autonomy on her mother. To the extent that she senses parental vulnerability, she may sacrifice independence to stay available. "Just as child incompetence may elicit parental caregiving, so may parental incompetence elicit child caregiving" (Cassidy & Berlin, 1994, p. 984). A daughter might deny or minimize her capacity for independence so as to remain available to her mother, thereby using her dependence to care for her mother.

> She may realize that heightened dependency and reduced exploration are at some level reassuring to the parent, [her] immaturity reassures the parent that she will be needed, [her] dependence reassures the parent that she will not become an adult and leave. (Bacciagaluppi, 1985, p. 371, cited in Cassidy & Berlin, 1994, p. 985)

An adolescent's continued dependence can offer security to a parent who lacks confidence in an attachment that is not ensured by continuing need. As a young woman becomes autonomous, her attachment to parents becomes more elective; she can now meet her needs on her own, through relationships outside the family. Attachment does not necessarily become any less genuine or strong when it is driven by a mutual wish for connection rather than need. A young woman's individuation and autonomy can enrich the lives of parents, not because they live vicariously through her or take pride in their success as parents, but because they gain from connecting to her as a person in her own right.

Therapists Cannot Escape the Pitfalls Associated with Attachment

Therapists are in a better position than parents to deal with the adolescent struggle with attachment. Obviously, their relationship with a patient is not as intense or longstanding. Even female therapists working with teenage girls will not experience feelings of symbiotic connection to the degree that a mother and daughter might. Yet, intense attachment can develop in therapy that may be experienced as a threat to the mother–daughter relationship. A young woman may experience this attachment and her wish to confide in a therapist as disloyal, and she may be reluctant to accept influence from another caregiver. Parents may fuel this negative reaction if they are uncomfortable with their daughter's connection to the therapist.

The treatment relationship, like the mother–daughter bond, has the potential to undermine autonomy rather than support it. Therapists can provide a launching pad for the adolescent, helping her to separate from regressive dependence on her parents and transition to meaningful attachments outside the family. But it is not always clear how a particular patient is using the treatment relationship and what she needs from the therapist at any time. Does she need to oppose therapeutic influence or attachment so as to manage feelings of disloyalty to her mother? In this case, resistance may allow her to protect her connection to her mother as she participates in therapy.

Therapists must question the meaning and impact of therapeutic attachment and modify their approach to the patient accordingly. Should they temper their attempts to establish an attachment because the therapeutic relationship is temporary, because they do not want to compete with the parent, or because they risk fostering excessive dependence? Is the patient resisting attachment because she needs to assert autonomy? And if so, does she need the therapist to continue to invite attachment so that she can demonstrate her independence by refusing it? Alternatively, does she need the therapist to step back and lower expectations for disclosure or contact? If she is afraid that she could become too dependent, should the therapist try to help her overcome this fear? Or, might the patient be more aware than the therapist of her susceptibility to regressive dependence? In short, behaviors that the therapist might regard as an obstacle to therapeutic work could, in fact, be serving to protect the level of independence that the patient has been able to achieve.

In the chapters to follow, I use composite case examples to explore these questions—questions that I ask myself throughout the course of any therapy with adolescent or young adult women. The questions will not be completely answered with any patient, and they must be revisited again and again as needs shift through the course of a treatment. A patient may, for example, need to retreat to regressive dependence on a therapist to prepare to become more immersed in peer relationships, which would eventually reduce her reliance on the therapist. Therapists must be mindful of the risks of regressive attachment in treatment. But they must also consider the risk that the adolescent's tie to her mother or her fear of dependence could hold her back from establishing the kind of therapeutic attachment that she needs to develop relationships with peers and maximize her capacity for autonomy.

Chapter 2

~

Embracing Resistance
and Building Attachment

*I*t had appeared that treatment was off to a good start for Audrey. An intelligent, charming young woman, she brought great resources to therapy but, at thirty-four years of age, had been largely unable to achieve even seemingly modest goals. As we started meeting regularly, she seemed initially encouraged that she might be able to use therapy to begin to fulfill her potential. Audrey recognized that for no apparent reason, she would fail to pursue what she wanted, and even when she did secure a desired date or freelance job—a testament to her personal appeal—she would become disillusioned and lose interest. She admitted that she could be too impatient or intolerant and had consequently sabotaged and walked away from valuable opportunities. However, she would critically evaluate herself only after the relationship or job had been lost. Racked with regret, she would acknowledge her responsibility and question whether her critical judgment had been too harsh. But in the midst of a struggle, she did not seem able to tap into this capacity for self-reflection and would remain convinced that her dissatisfaction was justified—until it was too late.

Despite her initial enthusiasm for the therapy, I suspected that Audrey would, at some point, find me to be inadequate as well. Although I could anticipate this problem, I did not know how to prevent the seeming inevitability that I too would be rejected. I doubted that she would continue to value the therapy as the work became more challenging or laborious. Further, I believed that her experience of overwhelming dissatisfaction would repeat even if I identified such a negative reaction as part of her self-defeating pattern. I felt tempted to placate Audrey and avoid confrontation to prolong her positive attitude. But more than that, I wanted to do everything possible to foster attachment, and to this end, I would try to tolerate and work with her limited capacity for frustration and commitment.

But I did not want to perpetuate dysfunction by tiptoeing around her critical attitudes or denying my own needs to avoid frustrating her. I feared that even if I did everything I could to accommodate her needs and expectations, Audrey might still choose to end treatment. I could not prevent her from repeating her tendency to abandon commitments, and if I pushed, it might drive her away more quickly. I needed to try to find a way to offer new experience within the constraints imposed by her resistance, which might allow her to make different choices in our relationship and eventually outside of treatment.

Repeating Dysfunctional Patterns in the Therapeutic Relationship

To fully understand her resistance to treatment, I needed to understand Audrey's fears and difficulties in her other relationships. Most recently, Audrey had been struggling with her failure to pursue a promising dating possibility with a man who frequented her regular coffee shop. Men found her attractive, but few sparked her interest, so the possibility of making a connection with someone with real appeal represented an important opportunity. Nonetheless, she would not strike up a conversation or even smile at him. She was preoccupied with this man, but in his presence, she masked her interest. When she would run into him, Audrey would inevitably leave the coffee shop plagued by the knowledge that she might have lost her last opportunity. Lacking any other means to contact him, she could never be sure when or if they would cross paths again.

Audrey had sought therapy because she had become so frustrated by failed efforts to build her life that she had become depressed. She felt hopeless and apathetic, deprived and cheated. After working with her for several months, I came to believe that Audrey had difficulty pursuing, and perhaps more importantly, sustaining her excitement about anything. She was a talented designer and had worked at top firms, but she would quickly grow frustrated with colleagues and managers. Even when she was assigned the highest profile, most creative projects, she would feel frustrated by the constraints or pressures imposed by the firm or the client. So after quitting a number of jobs, she began to work freelance. But even from a position in which she could exercise more control, she would eventually begin to feel frustrated and bored—a response that had prevented her from building positive business relationships and a thriving practice.

With men, Audrey had the capacity to feel attraction, but she was too critical, easily let down, and sensitive to potential rejection to pursue a mature relationship. Because she also had difficulty empathizing with another person, she was likely to experience his or her needs as an imposition. Although she longed for a romantic relationship, she was ambivalent about intimacy. The closeness and commitment she craved would soon intrude on her personal space and freedom. When she liked someone, she felt vulnerable, and she might have been quick to reject because she feared any critical response. Audrey possibly recognized that her current love interest would be most appealing from a distance—that she could be disappointed if they actually became involved. She might have resisted acting on her desire in order to protect a fantasy that would never be matched by actual experience.

Audrey initially seemed interested in exploring her self-defeating attitudes in therapy. But after several months, she began to complain that she was not changing quickly enough, and she began to cancel sessions sporadically. Like jobs and boyfriends that seemed more promising than they turned out to be, the therapy was proving to be a disappointment. She did not criticize me directly, but I suspected her cancellations reflected her fading investment. She was creating a self-fulfilling prophecy—her irregular attendance represented a form of resistance that could limit what we might accomplish, and it taxed my enthusiasm. Based on this experience with her, I began to understand one reason why her dating relationships might lose their spark. Audrey acknowledged that her frustration with therapy felt familiar, but she did not seem to recognize that her dissatisfaction could influence the other person and the course of their relationship. She believed that the right man or job was out there, and when she found them, she would no longer have to face the kind of frustration that tainted her current relationships.

To protect the treatment, I felt inclined to oppose or limit Audrey's increasing tendency to cancel. I wished for her to be more committed to the treatment, more patient, and more tolerant of inevitable frustration. I knew that I would not be able to convince her that treatment might make a meaningful difference in her life, even though it would likely be less than she hoped. My perspective would be easy to dismiss because I had a vested interest in her willingness to continue to participate and value the treatment. At moments, I questioned whether I was meeting Audrey's needs; after all, therapy had not yet enabled her to embrace any commitment, inside or outside of treatment. But she was contributing to the limitations of the therapy, and there was no reason to believe that she would be more able to sustain her investment if she worked with anyone else.

Rather than opposing her resistance, I wanted to understand it. Following her initial "attraction," she had begun to doubt my value, as she did with virtually all the men she had dated. However, I had more motivation and capacity to absorb her rejection than a boyfriend would. I did not get into a power struggle; I did not try to convince her of my point of view; and I remained engaged with her and eager to understand her experience of our relationship. I also recognized that her pattern of cancellations served defensive function, which helped me to stay engaged.

Audrey could reject me without losing our relationship. I tolerated her cancellations, in this way leaving the door open so that she could come and go as she pleased. The pattern of rejection and reunion escalated, from cancellations to actual breaks from treatment. On several occasions, she quit therapy and later retuned. Unlike a boyfriend, I was able to remain interested and available to pick up where we had left off. She could reflect on her dissatisfaction with treatment from a different perspective after she had left me, and here she had the chance to return. Her rejecting behavior did not doom her to unaddressable regret. The opportunity to resume our work allowed her to bring the insights that were triggered by loss back into our relationship. Repeating this experience over time, she might become able to feel the value of a relationship in the moment when she is frustrated. By holding onto both sides of her ambivalence, she might become able to maintain her attachment even as she recognizes the shortcomings and liabilities of the other person.

In therapy, Audrey could reject me without having to face the loss and regret she experienced when breaking up a dating relationship. I wondered whether I might be enabling her dysfunctional pattern by eliminating any significant consequence to her rejecting behavior. But a long history of painful loss had not served as a disincentive, and the opportunity to reflect when apart from me, while knowing that she could return, could represent a new experience and a possible pathway to change. Insight or confrontation would not eliminate Audrey's need to reject me, and so any therapeutic work would have to build from this rocky foundation. I was creating an opportunity to engage in a relationship that could survive her extreme ambivalence and could enable her to explore underlying feelings of vulnerability.

Working to Understand Rather Than Oppose the Patient's Resistance

Resistance was defined by *Webster's* dictionary in the 1950s as "opposition displayed by the patient to attempts of the analyst to penetrate the unconscious." In citing this definition, McLaughlin (1995) points out that this perspective, introduced by Sigmund Freud in the early 1900s, still prevails. We continue to recognize internal struggle, specifically the way that the patient is seen as resisting self-exploration and free association to ward off the emergence of painful or threatening unconscious memories, wishes, fantasies, or impulses. Mitchell and Black (1995) explain that Freud believed emotional experience may be dissociated because its content is "disturbing, unacceptable and in conflict with the rest of the person's ideas and feelings" (p. 4). The patient may oppose the therapist's efforts to bring these unsettling elements of her unconscious into consciousness.

Freud recognized the paradox of resistance: The patient would "strenuously ward off the efforts of the analyst to bring about the cure the patient sought" (McLaughlin, 1995, p. 96). But this does not mean that resistance is a bad thing or clinically counterproductive. McLaughlin (1995) explains that Freud saw "the enactment of these obstructive attitudes in the analytic relationship as inevitable and informative, and made their exploration and eventual verbal elucidation as forms of resistance indispensable to the therapeutic process" (p. 96). Indeed, from Freud's perspective, resistance is "not an obstacle to the treatment but the very heart of it" (Mitchell & Black, 1995, p. 8). Mitchell and Black (1995) explained the implications of Freud's thinking on the way in which therapists approach clinical work. Specifically, they should focus their efforts not on "circumventing" the patient's defenses to "discover her secrets," but rather on "exploring those very defenses as they manifested themselves in the analytic situation" (p. 8).

Although it may be used to defend against painful or unacceptable unconscious material, resistance is expressed in the context of a relationship: that is, the patient is opposing what the therapist is trying to do. In this sense, it is interpersonal and interactive. Fear or defiance in relation to a parent can be replayed with a therapist, and this transfer of attitudes from the past can become a source of resistance within treatment. Interpersonal theorists recognized that therapists also play a role in "augmenting or mitigating the patient's resistive behaviors" (McLaughlin, 1995, p. 105). Through the influence of their personality, their response to the patient, and approach to the treatment relationship, therapists participate in re-creating familiar patterns, both adaptive and dysfunctional.

Audrey's primary resistance took the form of cancellations. She persisted with this oppositional stance in the face of confrontation and was well aware that she was sabotaging her treatment. The gratification that Audrey derived from asserting control in this manner carried more weight than her motivation to take charge of her life. The stubborn and self-defeating nature of this behavior suggested that her resistance functioned, at least in part, to defy. She had achieved independence from family—she had a job, her own home, and friends—but Audrey had maintained a preoccupation with, and investment in, opposition. Although she was an adult, there was an adolescent flavor to this resistance. She would willfully sacrifice what she might know to be in her best interest for the gratification of asserting control.

This type of provocative resistance has its roots in adolescence, when the need to assert an independent identity is expressed through opposition. But like Audrey, young women may persist with defiant resistance into adulthood, as they continue to grapple with autonomy and control over their lives. The struggle to challenge authority—the fuel for normal teenage defiance—may continue to be evident in the therapeutic resistance of young adult women. There may be continuing need to transfer to the treatment relationship one's past and current struggle to emerge from dependence on the mother, to individuate and to assert autonomy. The young woman needs to rebel against parents and therapists to explore and assert ways that she is different from her caregivers, to forgo her own wishes for approval, and to maintain a separate emotional world. To this end, she may reject what the therapist offers, even though she knows she needs the help.

Teenagers are more likely to express resistance through action, often in the form of dramatic, provocative behavior that highlights their power to do what they want. Acting out also serves to defuse and distract from uncomfortable feelings that might be stimulated by therapeutic exploration. By relying on action to deal with distress, they may try to avoid depending on the therapist. But furthermore, they may be gratified by the thrill of defiance and the opportunity to release affect through reckless behavior. By adulthood, the intensity and drama of the acting out may diminish, and, as exemplified by Audrey's cancellations, tamer or more deliberate action may be used to defuse or oppose the clinical work.

A young woman may try to preserve childhood attachments even as they become increasingly maladaptive and ill suited to the demands and opportunities of her emerging adult life. Consequently, she may resist therapeutic pressure to relinquish familiar patterns. If the treatment relationship or therapeutic work is perceived as a threat to the patient's actual or internalized connection with her family, it will likely mobilize resistance. And if the patient fears that she will be unable to fend off threatening therapeutic influence, she may take flight from the treatment.

Dependent longings stirred by the transition to adulthood can fuel defensive efforts. Based on his work in a college mental health setting, Eichler (2006) described the way that passive–regressive wishes may be triggered by the pressure to manage independently from family, take on adult responsibilities, and confront personal limits. "Self-destructive and reckless behaviors may involve, in part, frantic efforts to maintain omnipotent defenses against the narcissistic injuries that are an inevitable part of finding one's place in the adult world" (Eichler, 2006, p. 31).

A young woman may need to approach therapy in a manner that minimizes her sense of vulnerability and dependence, even at the expense of exploring feelings and conflicts. She may be able to build and sustain a therapeutic attachment only if she has room to avoid, deny, or even act-out feelings that seem potentially over-whelming. Therapists can best support attachment and maximize potential for clinical exploration if they try to understand and accept the patient's fear and opposition.

Adaptive Functions of Resistance

Resistance is not merely opposition to therapy. It expresses aspects of the patient's sense of self, her approach to relationships, and internalized family influence. These longstanding patterns serve adaptive functions and therapists cannot necessarily antici-pate what will be lost if the patient makes a change. For this rea-son, it is essential for therapists to try to understand the role and value of any particular resistance. The effort to appreciate the patient's need to protect and preserve familiar patterns might par-adoxically enable the patient to feel sufficiently safe to consider letting go of defenses. I address here some adaptive functions of resistance. The following is not intended to be an exhaustive list, but rather to present the kinds of factors that a therapist might consider when confronted with defenses to therapeutic change. I have identified below some of the more common reasons why young women might resist therapeutic influence:

- To preserve attachments to family and familiar emotional and interpersonal patterns.

- To try to adhere to family and social expectations and values that may be at odds with one's identity.
- To pace attachment so as to avoid overwhelming dependence.
- To establish and assert autonomy.
- To protect against regret for opportunities that have been lost because of failure to change earlier.

Preserving Attachments to Family and Familiar Emotional and Interpersonal Patterns

Even if the patient recognizes that her attachments constrain her development, she might not be ready to let go of these sources of support. She may not yet have more functional alternatives. Further, she may not yet be able to even imagine the possibility of different experience with regard to relationships or her sense of self. By challenging dysfunctional attachments, therapists might be threatening an emotional lifeline—a connection that the patient cannot imagine being able to change or replace.

In the effort to promote healthier ways to deal with feelings and relationships, therapists may challenge the very strategies that protected the patient in childhood. For example, a therapist might encourage a young woman to open herself in ways that would have made her vulnerable to ridicule from parents or siblings. The patient may have needed to deny anger or sadness so as to avoid negative parental reactions or to protect a depressed parent. She may have learned to avoid conflict by watching the expression of anger spiral into rage, withdrawal, or damaging marital battles.

However, as a young woman's life moves beyond her family, the strategies that were adaptive in her childhood may interfere with her ability to embrace new experience. By late adolescence, a defense that developed in response to family stressors has often "outlived its usefulness and instead became an independent source of [her] difficulties" (Eichler, 2006, p. 26). Restricted affective expression, which may have been adaptive within a volatile family, may block intimacy with partners who, like the therapist, may be emotionally accessible. If a patient expects that others will respond like her parent(s), she may be unconsciously driven to relate in a manner that shapes her relationships to conform to old patterns, provoking familiar responses even with people who have more emotional capacity and tolerance. She may navigate toward partners who bear some similarity to her parents, then relate to them in a manner that heightens repetition at the expense of the opportunity that exists for new experience.

Dena came to therapy severely depressed, yet she denied any emotional vulnerability. Her flat, matter-of-fact presentation reflected an adaptation to a family that did not express or respond sensitively to feelings. Dena's parents, born and raised in the Philippines, struggled in their early life with poverty. Work was valued and emotional needs were regarded as self-indulgent. With little personal experience receiving emotional support, they most likely did not even think about Dena's feelings. Having immigrated as adults, they were unfamiliar with American culture. Consequently, as a child Dena did not fit comfortably with her peers, and she lost opportunity to derive support from social relationships.

Dena was accustomed to being self-sufficient, and even as she described suicidal thoughts and feelings of emptiness, she denied the need for emotional support. She cursed a lot, not to vent anger as much as to communicate that she was tough and invulnerable. In response to my direct questions, she denied any anxiety about entering treatment. Her only concern was whether I would be strong enough to deal with her and meet her needs.

Dena adopted a similarly defensive approach to relationships outside of therapy. She bragged that she could seduce any man in the bar that she frequented and have sex with him. She tallied these sexual encounters as "notches on her belt." Dena dismissed my concern about possible dangers, assuring me that she knows how to handle herself. She always uses a condom and plans escape routes to minimize risk—certainly good precautions—but she refused to acknowledge the reality that she could not control these men or prevent violence.

Because she was making self-protective efforts, I did not challenge Dena as I would, had her sexual behavior seemed motivated by overtly destructive intent. Moreover, I did not believe that I could persuade her to abandon these sexual exploits. I recognized the danger, but I did not want to impose pressure that might interfere with her ability to attach to me. By forgoing efforts to be immediately protective in favor of establishing a secure base of attachment, I hoped to provide emotional support that might reduce the drive toward promiscuity. I wanted to create opportunity for Dena to explore the feelings that motivated her behavior.

Attention to her emotional experience might satisfy some of the
need that fueled her sexual craving.

Therefore, rather than trying to influence her behavior
directly, I worked to understand Dena's need for the sexual liaisons. I asked about her experience with these men. She was eager
to talk about how and why she approached particular men, and
how she felt before, during, and after sex. On the surface, at least,
Dena felt proud of her ability to seduce, and my questions allowed
her to exhibit her bravado. As I listened, I recognized that Dena
was not really drawn to sex but rather was seeking conquest—the
thrill of going out and being able to pick up any man. She did not
just like the excitement; she *needed* it.

Dena had never talked about her sexual experience before, and
she appreciated my interest. Despite my concern about her behavior, I felt closer to her as I understood more about this part of her
life. Dena seemed to feel closer to me as well, and she began to reveal
more. I learned that her sexual expeditions were fueled by a desperate need to escape a sense of restlessness and emptiness. When
home alone at night, she would binge to try to fill up emotionally.
Both the compulsive bingeing and the pain of overeating would distract from her feelings. As with her sexual behavior, I responded to
reports of her binge episodes not by confronting her problems with
food or making a plan with her to manage her symptoms—which
would have introduced some pressure toward change—but by
exploring the feelings that triggered this behavior.

Because she was free from the need to protect her defensive
patterns, Dena could acknowledge that the sexual conquests
made her feel desirable and powerful. I did not judge her behavior, but I did challenge her belief that she was powerful in relation
to the men. I asserted that Dena could be in control only as long
as she was allowed to be—in fact, she was at the mercy of men
who could overpower and violate her. I was confronting her
denial, specifically her sense of invulnerability, without imposing
pressure to change. She explained that she would feel the high of
being desired when she seduced the man, and she enjoyed having
the power to gratify his longings. In the moment, Dena believed
that she could hang onto this feeling. But she acknowledged that
the thrill of the conquest would inevitably be fleeting. The
dreaded feelings of despair and worthlessness would return.

Dena's sexual behavior did not appear to be repeating any sort of childhood sexual abuse. Rather, she resorted to risk taking to distract herself from intolerable feelings that may have their origins in less tangible experiences of childhood vulnerability. She recalled being teased about her weight and clothes. As a child, she retained the dress and customs of her parents. Now as an adult, she could dress fashionably seductively, but she still avoided eye contact. She had not overcome this feeling of inadequacy and consequently still feared that she might see ridicule in the eyes of others.

Increased understanding of the feelings underlying her defensive patterns may or may not change Dena's behavior. As she made these insights, she continued her sexual liaisons. Yet, as she becomes more aware of her motives, she could potentially exercise more control over her choices and be more realistic about the implications of her behavior. Dena seemed to derive a sense of security from our relationship that allowed her to acknowledge some vulnerability. She admitted that emotional struggle drove her sexual behavior and that the conquest would provide an emotional boost, but only momentarily; the problem was temporarily alleviated, but not resolved.

Perhaps because of her growing attachment, Dena also seemed to be developing some identification with me. I noticed that several months into the treatment, she began to carry a knapsack that was similar to the one that I used. She seemed delighted when I noticed her bag and expressed my sense of connection with her. I had expressed concern about Dena's safety at times, but she seemed more attuned to my self-protective feelings. In the midst of one of her sessions, and with no connection that I could see to anything in our conversation, she pulled out a vial of antiseptic lavender lotion. She assured me that I would like this product and explained that she uses it to clean her hands when she is out, such as on the subway. She said she thought that I would like the fragrance and that I might want to be able to kill germs anywhere. I shared with her my enjoyment when I smelled her lotion and told her that I might buy some. With these small steps and moments of connection, our relationship was deepening and Dena was beginning to introduce something gentle and nurturing into her life, even as her defensive behavior persisted.

Trying to Adhere to Family and Social Values That May Be at Odds with One's Sense of Identity

A young woman may resist therapeutic exploration that has a potential to lead down a path that would conflict with family and social expectations and values. She may fear disapproval or rejection, a loss of stature, regard, or sense of connection. But perhaps even more, she may have internalized values that are in conflict with her own passions or inclinations. She may focus on the prospect of conflict with her family to avoid confronting her own internal conflict between what she thinks she should be doing in her life and what she is drawn to do.

Her wish to stay within the confines of what is valued and acceptable may prevent her from even recognizing points of divergence, and consequently she may resist looking inward to consider what, in fact, brings her pleasure, meaning, and fulfillment. Consequently, she may fail to explore her sexuality, alternate religious or political interests, or career options that would be regarded as less secure, worthwhile, or prestigious. When therapists try to help a young woman recognize and embrace parts of her identity that might be at odds with her family or social reference group, they must consider the impact on her actual and internalized connections, especially to parents.

Maureen was extroverted, lively, and popular. Since early adolescence she had dated a lot. She was heavily involved in sports, often competing or teaming up with boys, and she developed close friendships in this context that sometimes turned romantic. Late in high school, however, her relationship with her best girlfriend became sexual. She had never felt this intimate or excited before, but she considered the sexual part of their relationship to be mere experimentation. She was the youngest in a large Catholic family, and all her siblings were married with children, except an older brother who was studying to become a priest, so the notion of pursuing a sexual relationship with a woman was unthinkable. Maureen herself was deeply committed to her religion, and when she started at Boston College, she began dating guys again.

None of these relationships became serious, however, and Maureen would end them for various reasons. After college she again fell into a romantic relationship with a woman, Vivian, but this time sex was the main attraction. The relationship was immediately intense and passionate, and despite the differences in their background and education, Maureen became attached. Yet, she could not take the relationship seriously. She would never "date" a woman—and, moreover, Vivian drifted through temporary jobs, drank too much, barely spoke to her family—a lifestyle that was completely at odds with everything that Maureen valued. She would consequently pull away from Vivian, even for months at a time, but they would inevitably arrange to meet, have sex, and fall back into the relationship.

Vivian proved to be the first in a series of sexual relationships Maureen had with women, none of whom shared the base in friendship and common background that had characterized her relationships with her boyfriends. It was at this point that Maureen came to therapy. She was distressed by her attraction to women and her failure to be able to commit to and marry a man. She felt that her dalliance with women reflected a dark side to her sexuality that she was determined to suppress in the service of finding a "healthy" relationship with a man.

I believed Maureen's interest in women was more serious than she would acknowledge, but I was also aware that a same-sex romantic relationship was completely at odds with the religious beliefs, values, and expectations within her family and Catholic community. I think that Maureen expected me to discourage these sexual relationships with women who, in her mind, would have been wildly inappropriate partners even if they had been male. But I did not. I accepted that she wanted to marry a man and have children with him, but was attracted to women. In particular, I expressed interest in these intense sexual relationships, and I tried to explore with Maureen what she got from them and how they might even be fulfilling, in at least some respects, despite the obvious problems from her perspective.

I think that Maureen was most affected by my comfort with her sexual interest in women. She had kept it secret, and this was the first time she had ever talked about this part of her life. As Maureen began to accept the sexual part of these relationships, I began to wonder with her whether she might be choosing partners who are so different from her and, to some extent, less emotionally stable, not because she was drawn to the unpredictability and volatility, as she believed, but because she was afraid of becoming too serious—falling in love.

Several months later, Maureen began to develop a new friendship with a woman, Lilly, who had a history of committed sexual
relationships with women. As their relationship moved forward,
she complained that it lacked the passion that she had experienced in her past relationships. But the emotional connection was
undoubtedly deeper. Maureen believed that Lilly was a good person, but she was just not able to get sexually excited with her. I
believed that Maureen could not allow herself to experience emotional closeness together with sexual passion, because that might
mean that she might want a woman as her partner. She could tolerate her sexual interest only so long as she could keep it as a private, compartmentalized part of her life.

Lilly was undaunted by Maureen's ambivalence, and the relationship progressed. Maureen always talked with me about breaking up with Lilly, yet she continued to see more of her and even
introduced her as a "friend" to friends and family. She emphasized
that the relationship was limited because she could never disclose
its true nature. It would devastate her parents, her siblings, her
whole extended family and was at odds with her religion. I suspected that, given the extent of her attachment to family and their
central place in her life, she would be unable to sustain her bond
to Lilly if, in fact, her parents could not accept a same-sex relationship. But I believed that Maureen's real conflict was within
herself. She could not accept that she was sexually attracted to
women, and I thought, in love with Lilly. The more domestic and
less career oriented of the two, Lilly had even spoken of having a
child with Maureen, which she would be willing to stay home and
raise, allowing Maureen to pursue her more consuming career.
(This role choice might have been more of an issue with some of
the men that she had dated.)

I believed that Maureen was so preoccupied with anticipated
negative reactions of family and friends because she wanted a reason not to commit to Lilly. She resisted taking responsibility for
her own ambivalence. To define her sexuality differently from her
mother would introduce separation into her relationship with her
mother, who remained her closest attachment. She had limited
her life choices up to this point to try to allow her identity to continue to conform to what was familiar, valued, and expected
within her family and to be like them. She perhaps reasonably
feared that she might hurt, or even devastate, her mother. But by

allowing this concern to influence her life path, she would perpetuate a dysfunctional pattern in which she sacrificed her own needs to protect her mother.

Maureen was so emotionally attuned to, and connected with, her parents that she was able to find a way gradually, over the course of a few years, to help Lilly fit into her family. Parents and siblings related to her as Maureen's friend, which allowed them an opportunity to attach to Lilly before they needed to confront the issue of sexuality. Lilly left it up to them to deny or deduce, at their own pace over time, that there might be more to their relationship. Maureen was not out to challenge or defy the values of her family, she was just seeking acceptance. Her parents were likely well aware of her sensitivity to their opinions, and they seemed to decide, much to my relief, to keep any negative reactions or judgment to themselves. Her friends, who had also grown to love Lilly, seemed genuinely delighted as they recognized over time that they might become committed partners and that Lilly would consequently remain in their social circle.

In our dialogue, Maureen could explore her ambivalence, as I would voice what was probably one side of her feelings and she would voice the other. As she gradually saw that it was possible to find acceptance, she was more able to take ownership of her own intolerance. She also began to realize that she focused on Lilly's shortcomings, just as she did the imagined disapproval of her family, to set limits on the relationship—to find reasons not to move forward. As she was able to expand her identity to incorporate differences from her family, she became more able to embrace her sexual interest in women and create a place for Lilly in her life.

Pacing Attachment to Avoid Overwhelming Dependence

It can be difficult for therapists to sit back and accept the repetition of self-defeating patterns. Patients may be attached to behaviors or attitudes that interfere with their social and emotional development. A distressed adolescent girl is at particular risk for reckless sexual behavior, abuse of drugs, bingeing or purging, or other forms of potentially dangerous acting out. Depression or anxiety can cause her to retreat socially, and if this withdrawal is prolonged, she may lose connection to her peers. To prevent these negative repercussions, therapists may believe that it is vital for a young woman to develop a trusting alliance and embrace the therapeutic process as quickly as possible. When the cost of defensive behavior is high, therapists can lose sight of the adaptive function of resistance, which may increasingly seem like an obstacle that needs to be overcome.

A young woman may become more emotionally vulnerable as she lets go of defensive patterns that have provided a sense of security, contained threatening feelings, and enabled her to avoid more challenging interpersonal experience. She may also feel threatened by her growing therapeutic attachment. Consequently, she might need to resist or slow down the work or retreat from the therapeutic progress. Quite naturally, therapists might be inclined to oppose a patient's efforts to pull back from clinical work. Having witnessed progress, they may be eager to push further. In fact, the greatest danger may not be that therapeutic work will slow or even end prematurely (or what may seem premature to the therapist). Rather, it may be that the patient, fearful of disappointing the therapist, may push beyond her limits and become overwhelmed, losing gains that she has made.

Dr. M came to consult with me because her patient, Beverly, suddenly wished to terminate what appeared to be a successful and still vitally important treatment. The therapist feared that the patient's wish to end the work signaled treatment failure and that the premature termination could trigger destructive regression, reversing years of therapeutic work.

As I listened to her description of the course of treatment, I recognized that Dr. M had done a remarkable job of building an attachment with this young woman, whose anger and distrust had interfered with her ability to develop supportive relationships. Because of her therapeutic attachment, Beverly had become able, after several years of treatment, to resist acting on self-destructive impulses that had been habitual. She had not purged or cut her arms for more than a year and had begun to experience unprecedented stability. She was less needy and angry, and her relationships were becoming less volatile. Rather than engaging in destructive behaviors to manage painful feelings, she increasingly came to rely on Dr. M.

Through the first years of therapeutic work, Beverly had used deprivation and self-inflicted pain to deal with distress. Her anger and aggression, which were most often self-directed, had defended against hunger for love and acceptance. Dr. M was relieved when the patient stopped injuring herself, and she took this change as evidence that the therapy was on track. Beverly was becoming more able to deal with her feelings and longings by talking about them. In the absence of this acting-out behavior, her clinical work deepened. She began to describe painful childhood experiences that she had previously avoided. She became more dependent on the therapy to explore her experience and express feelings.

From this more emotionally expressive position, however, Beverly could no longer maintain the self-sufficient stance on which she had previously relied to contain dependent longings. She became more and more preoccupied with her therapist. She had fantasies of following Dr. M home or remaining in her office after the session had ended. She reported that she was having impulses to act destructively or precipitate a crisis to force Dr. M to become more involved with her.

Beverly talked about these fantasies in sessions and she did not act on them—also a remarkable accomplishment. But by disclosing her extreme attachment, she was making herself even more vulnerable. She was increasingly frightened by her dependence and the regressive wishes it stimulated. Although Beverly understood and respected the limitations of the therapeutic relationship, she began to feel more deprived. She came to resent anyone who might get more of Dr. M than she did, such as the therapist's children, and she felt guilty about resenting Dr. M, whom she loved. Dr. M, however, was not threatened by Beverly's expression of resentment and longing. In fact, she welcomed the opportunity to explore these reactions and their roots in childhood deprivation as a means to help Beverly better tolerate feelings of dependence.

Beverly knew that her therapist was proud of the progress that she had made. She likely feared that Dr. M would feel disappointed or disillusioned if she lost control over her impulses, and she believed that she was on the verge of doing so. She restrained herself from taking destructive action and instead decided to take a break from treatment. When discussing her plans with her therapist, she downplayed her fear of losing control and emphasized her desire to live "closer to nature." She explained that she hoped to move away for 6 months or a year.

Dr. M was deeply committed to the treatment and aware of the patient's continuing clinical need. She knew that if Beverly left treatment, she might not return to deal with the issues they were currently addressing. The work had already yielded so much benefit that it seemed that further change was within reach. Dr. M regarded Beverly's plan as resistance, a means of avoiding the difficult issues that were emerging in the treatment. She wanted Beverly to express her resentment and fears, including her struggle with the limitations of the therapeutic relationship.

As I explored the course of the treatment with Dr. M, I began to think there might be wisdom in the patient's inclination to retreat—she may know better than Dr. M that she had reached a limit as to what she could tolerate. Beverly might have needed to create distance from her therapist to contain her longings. But even if her feelings toward Dr. M had become overwhelming, I did not think that it necessarily suggested therapeutic failure. Dr. M had recognized from the outset that attachment would be threatening to Beverly, and she tried to pace the development of their relationship accordingly. She had tolerated Beverly's efforts to resist treatment, at least up to the point that she wanted to quit. It is possible that Beverly's overwhelmed reaction was inevitable, given the kind of therapeutic progress that she had made.

The opportunity to take leave from the treatment, although extreme as a defensive measure, could represent a means to contain potentially destructive, regressive impulses and protect therapeutic gains. If Dr. M supported Beverly's decision to end treatment, she could better preserve the therapeutic connection and maximize the possibility that the patient might return (if and when she felt more able to manage dependent longings) or might seek treatment from a therapist in her new community.

Dr. M's wish to continue the treatment might have overwhelmed Beverly's defenses. Given Beverly's attachment and her wish to please, therapeutic disapproval might have made her feel too conflicted to be able to stop treatment when she needed. To please her therapist, Beverly might have pushed past her limits and regressed to self-destructive behavior, losing some of the ground she had gained. Even if Beverly were stopping prematurely, in the sense that she could in fact go at least a bit further in therapy, the progress that she had already made could nonetheless endure, and the therapy would still have greatly enhanced her life.

Resistance as an Expression of Autonomy

A young woman may explore and assert her independent identity by challenging or defying her therapist. Treatment may offer opportunity to question authority and rebel in a manner that might not have been possible within the family. If therapists are more able than parents to tolerate such challenge, they can create a forum within which to work through problems encountered as the patient tries to assert autonomy within a caregiving relationship.

An adolescent may persist with risky and self-defeating behaviors in the face of therapeutic confrontation. Rebellious behavior in treatment can be disappointing, disturbing, or, if dangerous, even frightening to the therapist, who may be tempted to try to rein in the acting out by attempting to manage whatever appears to be overwhelming to the adolescent. This clinical stance reflects the notion that self-defeating or destructive behavior may represent deficient coping capacity or inability to manage feelings and impulses.

Yet, this self-defeating behavior may be part of a normative, highly conflicted struggle to separate from close bonds with family, especially the mother. By hurting or defeating herself, the adolescent can rebel without actually carving out a viable niche in the world that could free her from dependence on her parents. Similarly in psychotherapy, the patient can rebel by rejecting therapeutic influence. She acts defiantly but in a manner that seems to heighten her need for therapeutic support. This resistant behavior therefore expresses both sides of the conflict between autonomy and dependence.

Self-defeating, defiant behavior should not be regarded solely as a manifestation of regression or as a permanent or fixed adaptation. Rather, it may be part of an evolving struggle with autonomy that includes progressive strivings. I am not suggesting that adolescent defiance is necessarily self-defeating in nature, and I am not suggesting that self-defeating behavior is necessarily healthy or adaptive for young women. Rather, the provocative or self-defeating nature of defiance may disguise an underlying progressive struggle. The patient may be using apparently regressive, defiant behavior to begin to explore and assert her autonomy.

If therapists view such acting out only as regressive, they will be more inclined to try to exert control—an effort that is likely to fuel the patient's drive to defy. It can further undermine the adolescent's own sense of responsibility for her choices. The stage is then set for her to assert her autonomy by resisting the therapist's protective efforts. The patient's independent strivings may be lost in the resulting power struggle. She can deny her fear and ambivalence regarding autonomy, indulging reckless impulses while relying on the therapist to take a protective stance and assume responsibility for the clinical work.

For some young women, resistance may mark a departure from a history of compliance or passivity. By defying or challenging, they risk frustrating or disappointing their therapist. Fear of encountering a critical response can inhibit the expression of autonomy. Therefore, the willingness to disappoint a therapist may be a prerequisite for independent decision making. However, efforts to exercise autonomy must be differentiated from efforts to provoke negative reactions in the service of denying longings for approval. The former may be progressive and the latter regressive, and it may be difficult for the therapist to know which is being played out at a given time.

Defiance may also function to assert difference from the therapist, which can be part of the process of exploring and defining one's independent values, preferences, and viewpoint. But if the patient is to thoughtfully differentiate herself from her therapist, her defiance must be selective. Resistance may lose its adaptive value if it becomes ubiquitous. When the patient is caught in the need to oppose, she is not exercising independent thought any more than if she were motivated by an approval-seeking need to comply. When an adolescent automatically or consistently opposes the therapist, she may be avoiding the challenge of developing her own perspective. Therefore, a shift within treatment from consistent compliance to defiance may signal neither regression nor progression but rather an ongoing abdication of responsibility for independent decision making.

When therapists resort to exercising professional authority, in some way saying "You must participate in this treatment" or "You must stop this behavior," they are denying the limits of their power. Therapists cannot impose control unless the patient allows them to do so. But even if they could, and even if they were correct in assuming that the targeted resistance was in fact regressive or destructive, which it may not be, therapists might do more harm than good by compromising the patient's sense of autonomy. When therapists set limits based on their own capacity to tolerate a particular behavior or risk, they are not so much trying to control the patient as trying to protect themselves within the context of the treatment. However, when a therapist tries to break through resistance for the patient's clinical benefit, the patient could feel defeated and resort to more insidious or dangerous acting out to reassert her control. To this end, she might indulge in secret episodes of bingeing or purging or other reckless or destructive behaviors. Or she might appear to comply, changing a particular problematic behavior or attitude, while she, in fact, becomes emotionally closed to therapeutic influence.

When therapists assert power or authority, they may be able to influence the patient's thinking and choices. If this assertive behavior is a departure rather than the therapist's typical pattern, then the dominant position may introduce new experience and possibly expand the range of clinical interaction. Moreover, if there is a playful element to the interaction, which includes shared awareness that the patient is *allowing* the therapist to exert dominance, it could represent a means to explore power and submission. But if therapists consistently dominate or oppose resistance in a heavy-handed manner, they could create a polarization in which they are seen as being responsible for the patient. In the extreme, therapists can set up an expectation that they will step in to rescue. Whatever benefits might be conferred by efforts to break through a defense could be outweighed by cost for the young woman's sense of autonomy.

Resistance to Change as a Defense against Regret

Change forces an awareness of loss. When a patient contemplates breaking with dysfunctional patterns, she may envision not just the effort or struggle, but also the opportunities that might become available. To embrace the potential of new experience, however, she must face the cost of her longstanding, self-defeating attachments. In other words, to pursue new opportunities, she must acknowledge the losses she had sustained by past failure to do so, for example, the exploration that was precluded by her rigidity. Yes, it is wonderful to consider new possibilities, but what if she had pursued them earlier? Where would she be now? Would her life have taken a different and perhaps more fulfilling direction? Rather than motivating change, therefore, awareness of missed opportunities may drive resistance. As long as she continues to participate in dysfunctional patterns, a young woman does not have to confront feelings about the possibility that she could have freed herself sooner.

Despite their youth, some doors have already closed or seem to be closing for these patients. By the later adolescent years, decisions begin to shape one's adult life. Dysfunctional patterns begin to cost more, and it is not always possible to compensate for lost opportunities. Eichler (2006) discussed this issue in the context of his work with college students, addressing a problem that becomes exacerbated when the adolescent leaves school to face the commitments of adulthood:

> As one moves through late adolescence, with every choice made, other possibilities begin to recede: Selecting one major effectively rules out all others. Applying to medical school makes it less likely that one will go to law school or become a journalist or painter. Committing to a particular partner requires, at least for the time being, bypassing other liaisons and love possibilities. Moreover, with every choice, time passes. As young as they are, college students commonly complain of "falling behind" or having "wasted too many years." (p. 36)

As a young woman travels further down any path, it becomes more difficult to make a change. She encounters practical as well as emotional obstacles. It will likely be more challenging to go back to school after launching a career, for example, than it would have been to change majors while still in college.

Nonetheless, a young woman may believe her options are more limited than they, in fact, are. She may use the notion that it is "too late" defensively to avoid the risk that she could fail if she took on new challenges. If she follows her passion, she might face a more uncertain or difficult course. And if in doing so, she would be leaving a path chosen at least partly to please her parents, then she would face the risk of disappointing them. Change could also mean forgoing the fringe benefits of a path that is not as emotionally fulfilling. For example, it may be difficult to give up material success, which also affirms one's value, to follow a passion that might not provide as much financial freedom or security. Life may also be more difficult without the emotional or financial support from family. Consequently, fear of losing family backing may reinforce a young woman's inclination to continue to accommodate parental expectations and maintain the status quo rather than risk disrupting this connection. It can be easier to decide that change is not possible than to take on these risks and challenges.

A young woman may be frustrated by her late start and the fact that she now lags behind those who got on "the path" earlier in their lives. She might never be where she could have been, had she taken the supposed right direction from the outset. Her anger about what she has missed may interfere with her ability to embrace opportunities that become available. Regret about the road not taken is more abstract and therefore might be more tolerable than the regret she would feel if she actually tried to pursue her dream and found that she was falling short. To embrace current opportunity, one must mourn what has been lost. Mistakes and missed opportunities cannot be undone. When a young woman avoids pain by denying the loss or the possibility of change, she limits her present and future life.

As I mentioned when I introduced Audrey at the beginning of this chapter, by the time she entered therapy, she had already missed out on important opportunities. She had rejected many devoted boyfriends and other possibly wonderful partners. Audrey would not invest enough to build solid commitments and more fully develop her potential and the potential of her relationships. Her reluctance to give up a view of people (including me) as ultimately disappointing served to protect her from recognizing all that she had already lost. She could still build a loving romantic relationship, but whatever she does now cannot retrieve what she had already squandered. Audrey had had a special connection with several of the men she had dated, who genuinely cared about her, and these relationships could be not revived.

Audrey tended to blame others for her failure to get what she needed. To break from this pattern, she would have to recognize the magnitude of the loss and take responsibility. By withdrawing her investment from relationships and commitments when frustrated and doubtful, she had sacrificed much that was precious and unique. If she pushed herself to continue to invest in therapy even when she felt frustrated by what she perceived as her lack of progress, she would be forced to consider what might have happened in other relationships and ventures had she persisted.

Although she was able to see that her withdrawal from therapy repeated the pattern that she was seeking to change, this insight did not impact her inclination to cancel. Audrey's sense of herself and relationships was centered on the certainty that she would be disappointed. To change, she would need to challenge her view of the course of her life, and she could not bear to think that she could have achieved different results by making different choices. In this way, anger and regret can become an obstacle for the therapeutic progress.

Embracing the Patient's Attachments

Therapists can begin to connect with an adolescent by embracing her attachments to her family and to familiar emotional and relational patterns. By accepting resistance in the service of protecting these attachments, therapists may provide a secure therapeutic base. This approach builds comfort and trust, and can allow for deeper clinical exploration and a better relationship in the long run. As I discuss in Chapter 4, as therapeutic attachment solidifies and the patient's emotional and relational experience expands over the course of treatment, a young woman may become more prepared to embrace change. Therapists might then have more room to challenge resistance and broaden therapeutic exploration without destabilizing the treatment.

Chapter 3

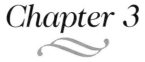

When Parents Collude
with Their Daughter's Resistance

Sylvia appeared to be mature for a fifteen-year-old, but she was vulnerable to criticism. I suspected that she could attach to me only so long as she could secure my approval, so I was unsure whether she would ally in a manner that could allow for challenge. Unfortunately, a few months into treatment, I learned that Sylvia was "hanging out" with adult men at an ice cream shop on a college campus near her high school, and consequently I felt forced to confront the risky nature of her behavior. She was seeking attention and trying to engage in conversation in order to entice one of the men who frequented the shop, most likely a college student, to sit with her. She longed to feel accepted (which she did not with her peers at school). I do not think that Sylvia or any of the young men who approached her necessarily wanted to have a relationship. But I feared that the man's interest could be based on sexual attraction and hers on a desire for personal acceptance. I was concerned that some young man might see the conversation as a prelude to sex. So far, Sylvia had made no physical contact, nor did she want to, but it seemed that she might be flirting in a manner that could communicate that she was more interested and prepared for sex than she really was.

I expressed concern about her safety, which I knew she would likely interpret as criticism. I could not be certain of the actual risk that Sylvia faced. It seemed possible that she was provoking more concern than might be warranted, but I was reluctant to withhold my feedback. Even if our attachment was not yet sufficiently resilient to absorb a critical response, I feared it would be negligent, especially given her young age, to ignore risks that she might not fully appreciate.

My confrontation seemed to damage her trust. Perhaps because she continued to feel angry and hurt, Sylvia provoked a second confrontation by bothering someone in my waiting room. Her behavior made me angry, especially because it impacted one of my patients. I felt that I had no choice but to set a limit regarding her behavior in my common space. Although I wanted to explore her feelings about my reactions and understand why she behaved as she did, Sylvia ended the therapy.

I had known the risks of criticizing Sylvia, and it was possible that I had overreacted to either or both of these provocations, but I think Sylvia had been determined to ignite my concern and ire. She resisted treatment by provoking a response from me that she could not tolerate, which gave her a reason to end therapy without having to feel that she was quitting. In this way, it seemed possible that our conflict might have been fueled by resistance to treatment. Sylvia had come to therapy because she had difficulty managing the stress of school, where she often felt socially rejected. But rather than talking about her hurt or loneliness, or questioning her social skills, she denied any distress, blamed her peers for her frustrations, and sought approval from older guys. Sylvia wanted to avoid confronting her social problems because it felt too painful.

It was also possible, however, that her parents were playing a role in Sylvia's resistance to treatment. They did not support my efforts to encourage Sylvia to reflect on her interpersonal impact or to take responsibility for her lack of social skills. Instead, they reinforced the idea that I was being inappropriately critical and that the other kids at school were immature, and in this way they fueled her inclination to blame others for her problems. For their own emotional reasons, which I, as Sylvia's therapist, was not in a position to understand or explore, Sylvia's parents did not want to acknowledge their daughter's social and emotional difficulties or support a therapeutic process.

Parental resistance can undermine therapeutic work with teenagers, and such opposition can be difficult to address particularly when a therapist is working individually with an adolescent. Parents might need their own treatment to be able to work out conflict they may have regarding their daughter's growing autonomy. When therapists are working individually and allied with the adolescent, they may not be able to talk as freely with parents. A young woman who is seeking her own separate therapy may be uncomfortable with contact between her therapist and her parents (even if she trusts the therapist's ability to protect her privacy). It may also be uncomfortable for the therapist to access information about the parents that the daughter does not know, that her parents might not want her to know, or that the therapist does not know that the daughter knows.

With these complications, it can be difficult for one therapist to address both an adolescent's individual clinical needs and those of the parents, and to deal with parental resistance to a daughter's individual therapeutic work. Consequently, therapists first need to think about whether they can work with an adolescent individually, or whether (and how) her parents or the whole family should be involved. Moreover, even within the context of an individual treatment, therapists must consider the role of parents in a patient's resistance. And more generally, therapists must consider how they will deal with parental reactions and influence on a daughter's therapy. To this end, they might need to consider the following questions:

- *Where should therapists draw boundaries in their work with an adolescent?* If a teenager is not ready to form an attachment or work on emotional issues independently, or if parents cannot support a daughter's separate ventures, then family therapy or conjoint parent–daughter treatment might be necessary. Perhaps family therapy could also serve as a precursor to individual psychotherapy. On the other hand, individual therapy might be appropriate from the outset if the adolescent seems to be ready to make use of a therapeutic relationship that is separate and private from her parents.

- *How should therapists deal with parental resistance that might surface over the course of treatment?* The family or conjoint approach would allow therapists to address their concerns directly. When working exclusively with the daughter, therapists might recommend alternative support for parents and might also help their patient to deal with therapy on her own terms, perhaps enabling her to resist the temptation to take on her parents' viewpoint.
- *How can a therapist tell whether an adolescent's resistance to treatment expresses her own opposition or parental reservations?* It can be difficult to determine the source of resistance. A daughter might provoke her parents to react negatively to her therapy because she does not want to take responsibility for her own opposition. Alternatively, she might resist change that threatens her parents out of a sense of loyalty.

Later in this chapter, I describe the way that these issues arose in my work with Sylvia. In particular, I focus on the role that parents might have played in Sylvia's resistance and in the ultimate demise of her treatment.

The Role of Parents and Family Loyalty in Resistance

Teenagers who are living with parents and are emotionally dependent on them may have the most difficulty tolerating therapeutic influence, particularly when it challenges or conflicts with parental influence. Even when a daughter resists parental input, their skepticism can dampen her investment in therapy, whereas their support may help her weather frustration and injuries in the work. Therapeutic progress that threatens the status quo within the family can trigger a withdrawal of parental support at a critical juncture, possibly undermining the daughter's commitment to therapy.

An adolescent may use parental ambivalence to cover her own negative reactions to therapeutic challenge. It is normal for parents to have reservations regarding change, and it is not necessarily a problem for therapy. But a daughter may, for defensive reasons, provoke her parents to question her treatment. She may stoke parental doubt, acting on her own resistance by mobilizing their opposition. Consequently, treatment can be threatened by forces that appear to be outside of the patient's control, but really may not be.

When resistance originates from family or when parents become the mouthpiece for the daughter's negative reactions to treatment, therapists are left in a difficult position. If they take a stand that is in opposition to that of the parents, the patient might be caught between their conflicting perspectives—a conflict that the therapist is likely to lose. If therapists are not working directly with parents, they may be unable to explore and work through their conflict or identify the patient's role in fomenting negative parental reactions. The therapist then has less leverage with which to confront the patient's resistance.

Certainly, therapists are in a better position to deal with parental concerns when parents are included in the treatment and therefore more able to explore their reactions to therapeutic progress. Such family-based intervention can reduce the risk that parents will undermine a daughter's treatment. Parents may be more supportive when they feel connected to the therapist. But if this connection depends on ongoing contact, it can compromise the therapist's ability to offer the adolescent an attachment that is independent and separate from her family.

If parents ultimately pull their daughter out of treatment, it does not necessarily mean that the therapy was unproductive. In fact, therapy may end because the patient made so much progress that the degree of change became too threatening to the parents or the adolescent. Once parents become caught up in the daughter's ambivalence, neither the daughter nor the therapist may be able to reverse the pressure to terminate. An adolescent and her family may be prepared to go only so far with a therapy at a given time. What looks like a therapist's failure may in fact reflect the emergence of overwhelming resistance from the patient and/or her parents, signaling the limits of their capacity to tolerate change at a given point in time. When parents and the daughter join together in opposing therapy, former sources of conflict within the family may be dismissed as they temporarily unite in their anger or skepticism.

Creating Boundaries from Parents in Therapy

Therapists may face conflict between creating a treatment relationship with an adolescent that is separate from her parents and accommodating the parents' wish to stay in touch with their daughter's treatment and possibly offer input. It is understandable that parents may want to know from the therapist how their daughter is doing, how she is using the therapy, and whether she is dealing with issues of concern to them, particularly because they may get little information directly from her. However, the adolescent may need privacy and the freedom to engage in a therapeutic relationship on her own. She may trust the therapist only to the extent that she can control what, if any, information gets back to her parents. The patient will likely feel freer to attach to a therapist if she thinks that the therapist likes and respects her parents, and will neither, on the one hand, ally with her against her parents or, on the other hand, take up take up her parents' agenda and become an agent for them.

Family influence and loyalty may also be internalized and may thereby influence a young woman's approach to therapy, even if she enters into an entirely separate and private individual treatment. The daughter may feel guilty about her attachment to the therapist or her exploration of her negative reactions to family. She may fear that her family will disapprove of changes and, in the extreme, withdraw love and support.

Pauline was highly motivated in therapy but fearful of the impact of change on her family. She came to therapy because she knew that she was sabotaging her dating relationships. She wanted to marry but feared that to do so would be to abandon her sister. Consequently, in recent years she had barely dated. As twins, the sisters had always been particularly close, and after their mother died when they were young teens, they had learned to rely on and care for each other. They were best friends and shared many entanglements, including their condominium. Pauline's sister had no desire to marry and was content with their current arrangement, whereas Pauline craved intimacy outside the family.

Pauline knew that her sister might criticize any man she dated, and she further knew that she was sensitive to her sister's opinion. She could not help but take on her sister's doubts, and so any negative feedback could undermine her affection and interest, causing her to withdraw from her boyfriend and eventually reject him. Whenever she complained to me about her sister's possessive nature, she felt guilty. In this way, her commitment to her sister became a source of resistance. Pauline focused on her sister's dependence rather than her own. Her preoccupation with family ties and obligations could be used to avoid a romantic relationship and all its emotional peril.

Parents' Resistance Can Undermine a Daughter's Therapy

I introduced Sylvia in the beginning of this chapter because she well exemplifies the problems that arise when parental resistance to treatment and conflict between parents and a therapist cannot be effectively addressed or teased apart from the patient's reactions to the therapy. Although I was working with Sylvia individually and she approached therapy independent of her parents (interviewing me on her own), I was concerned about parental reactions and opinions from the outset. We had all agreed that I would proceed with an independent treatment, but Mr. F, who worked from home and was primarily responsible for Sylvia, seemed to have difficulty allowing his daughter to deal with treatment apart from him. He remained actively involved behind the scenes, checking in with her about each session and voicing reactions.

Mr. F expected to have significant influence over the course of the therapy, without being directly involved. He wanted Sylvia to operate independently in therapy, but he also had opinions about what she needed. Specifically, he wanted me to help Sylvia with stress management to alleviate what he described as persistent problems with irritable bowel syndrome, insomnia, and teeth grinding. Perhaps to emphasize that that his parenting was not to be faulted, Mr. F explained that Sylvia's two older brothers were now happily married and professionally successful. It seemed that he could not tolerate the idea that his children could have emotional problems. Based on his approach to Sylvia's treatment, it appeared that Mr. F might not be comfortable with emotional expression or exploration. In the therapy, I wanted to try to provide a safe haven for Sylvia to express feelings in a manner that she might not be able to do at home.

I was not sure that Sylvia was ready for her own treatment, especially because she could get caught in a split between her father and me. The seeds had already been planted for Mr. F to pull Sylvia out of therapy if I did not follow his agenda or if the therapy stirred up too many feelings. Had Sylvia's parents been amenable, I might have been able to address family-based resistance by working with them together with Sylvia. But Mrs. F traveled extensively for work, making her largely unavailable, and I did not feel confident that I would be able to work with Mr. F, even if he were willing to participate. I also thought that it was possible that Sylvia might have more capacity to deal with feelings than her father did, and that she might be able to handle an individual therapy without parental support. And if I worked individually with Sylvia, there was a chance that I could help her become more independent of her father's influence. Therefore, despite the potential pitfalls, particularly the risk that her father might undermine the treatment, I decided to go the route of individual psychotherapy.

Once we started meeting, Sylvia quickly began to attach to me. Perhaps because of her limited contact with her mother, she seemed hungry for my attention and approval—she would frequently seek assurance that I thought she was special. I acknowledged my genuine affection and regard for her, but I also explained that her pressure for particular feedback made it difficult for me to spontaneously share my feelings. As Sylvia described her school experience, I learned that she put pressure on peers as well. She would intrude into their interactions, directly seeking immediate acceptance. When she was not included in a conversation or activity, she would feel angry and rejected and would devalue the other kids, explaining to me that they "weren't worth her time."

Sylvia seemed to have difficulty noticing and deciphering social cues that could potentially help her to approach others with more sensitivity. Cognitive or learning problems may have played a role, possibly exacerbating her social awkwardness. But Sylvia's failure to attune to the feelings and needs of others likely also reflected an emotionally based tendency to be self-absorbed. She did not tolerate frustration well, and when others did not provide what she wanted she would not hesitate to push back. Moreover, I think she felt lonely and deprived, and the associated frustration and anger might have driven her to approach interactions aggressively.

Sylvia may have alienated her peers because of her failure to recognize and respect boundaries. She did not seem to grasp the need for personal space—she would stand too close to others and speak too loudly. This behavior felt aggressive. I found myself backing away when we interacted in the waiting room, yet she did not seem to notice my discomfort. It is possible that she did not pick up on my nonverbal signal (e.g., moving back). But she might have also been determined to force the closeness she wanted, even if she knew I wanted more distance. I suspected that her vulnerability did not show in her social interactions, which could have made her less sympathetic or appealing. Her preoccupation with her own needs interfered with any empathic capacity she might have had.

Given her difficulty picking up on nonverbal communications and responding to the needs of others, it was not surprising that Sylvia was a loner at school. She had a few girlfriends, who were also socially marginal. Because these girls seemed to be as self-absorbed as Sylvia, their connections with each other were not particularly strong. They provided companionship but little emotional support. Sylvia connected best with teachers who, like me, would be less impacted by her failure to tune into their needs and more likely to appreciate her intellectual abilities and her wish for approval.

As long as I remained sympathetic to her frustrations and validated her perspective, Sylvia seemed eager to ally and even idealize me. I felt some pressure, for example, to agree with her conviction that her school had little to offer her socially. I did agree that the environment seemed competitive, but I also suggested that we might work on helping her learn better ways to make friends. Specifically, I noted that she does not give time for relationships to develop, or to allow others to approach at their own pace. Sylvia seemed to tolerate listening to my feedback, but she did not take it in. She remained attached to her self-protective belief that most kids in her school were not as mature as she was. Throughout this initial "honeymoon" phase of the treatment, Sylvia's father stayed in the background and continued to support the therapy.

As Sylvia began to express a greater range of feelings, she

seemed a bit more accessible and approachable. She began to talk more openly about her inability to break in socially at school and her difficulty relating to other kids. It was at this point that she revealed her habit of seeking interaction with men at the ice cream shop. These college-age men were more likely to respond to her overtures than a teenage boy might be. In this context, she may have appeared more confident than aggressive, and over the course of such time-limited interaction, her social limitations and emotional immaturity may have been less apparent. But most important, perhaps, the men who would respond to Sylvia might have interpreted her attention as a sexual invitation, and the resulting interaction might therefore have had different meaning to them than to her. If they responded, she would join them to talk and snack together.

Sylvia craved companionship and attention. With young adult men, she could stimulate interest that she did not get in school. I suspected from her description and tone that Sylvia was initiating contact by behaving seductively—perhaps showing her attraction or flattering them—and she was quite physically mature and sexually developed. It was possible that Sylvia was emphasizing the erotic flavor of the interaction to impress or provoke me. But I did become concerned that her flirtation might elicit a sexual response. Given her assertive demeanor, it would be easy for a man to think she was an adult. And because she could be oblivious to nonverbal cues and social signals and unaware of her interpersonal impact, she could be caught off guard if the interaction turned more sexual than she expected or intended. Although she might flirt to attract attention, she was probably not seeking sexual interaction, nor was she prepared for it.

I felt that I must confront the danger that one of these men could misinterpret Sylvia's behavior and make unwanted sexual advances. I hoped that Sylvia might share my concern if she saw her behavior the way that I did, yet I was also mindful that she had been unable to accept my perspective regarding her social behavior at school. Nonetheless, I wanted to try to make her more aware of what she might be communicating. Sylvia needed to be more cognizant of the signals that she might be giving in all of her interactions, but particularly with adult men. I did not believe that Sylvia and I disagreed about how much risk was acceptable. Rather, I thought that she might not be aware of the risk that she might be taking and how her behavior might be interpreted by a man.

My decision to confront Sylvia was primarily motivated by concern about her safety, but I had been looking for some leverage to address her empathic failures and insensitivity to social signals. With few friends, Sylvia had minimal opportunity to practice and develop relational skills and deal with her peers. I had been eager to break into this cycle, but I feared that critical feedback could jeopardize her attachment to me. When I confronted her inappropriately flirtatious behavior, Sylvia recognized that I wanted to protect her, but she nonetheless felt injured.

Sylvia complained to her father about my critical feedback, and he immediately sided with his daughter. In the next session Sylvia said that her father was not concerned about the men in the ice cream shop. He thought that I was "overreacting." I had seldom before been in a position in which I was more concerned than the parent about a teenager's behavior. Typically, I field calls from worried parents and help them to tolerate risk behavior in the service of supporting their daughter's autonomy and communicating trust for her judgment. But Sylvia had been able to enlist her father's support for her position in our conflict.

Mr. F might have legitimately had a different take on Sylvia's behavior with men. However, I think he took this opportunity to criticize me because he was increasingly opposed to the direction I had been taking in the treatment, specifically the fact that Sylvia had been expressing more feeling, particularly anger and frustration. Perhaps to be loyal and allied with her father, Sylvia would concede nothing to my point of view. However, I picked up hints that she was becoming a bit more careful and restrained in subsequent interactions at the ice cream shop.

Sylvia did not seem to want to acknowledge that I could influence her. I could not be sure whether she was using her father to support her own wish to dismiss uncomfortable feedback or whether she had turned to her father to give him the ammunition she knew that he wanted to discredit me. Regardless of her motive for pulling her father into our conflict, she could not side with me over him. Although she continued to attend sessions regularly and talk about her daily life struggles, Sylvia became more distant and less affectionate. Now she was less receptive to any feedback I might offer, on any topic. Not only did

Sylvia no longer idealize me, but she was becoming skeptical, even devaluing. She was beginning to dismiss me, as she did with kids at school who hurt her.

My relationship with Mr. F also seemed to deteriorate from tense to openly distrustful. Sylvia had amplified the split that had existed between us. According to Sylvia, we had taken opposing positions regarding her behavior, and she was caught between two of her caregivers. If Sylvia were to recognize my concern as protective rather than as unwarranted criticism or overreaction, she would be confronted with the possibility that her father might not be sufficiently protective, or at least not as much as I was. To be loyal to her father and to safeguard her sense that he could adequately protect her, she had to discredit me and this had a cost for my relationship with her and with her father.

When another conflict arose about one month later, my relationship with Sylvia had still not recovered. In this case, however, I was personally impacted by her behavior because the incident took place in my office space. The patient that I saw after Sylvia reported to me that Sylvia had lingered in the waiting room and persistently asked her personal questions. Then she sat and stared while my patient tried to avoid conversation. Sylvia had missed or, more likely, had chosen to disregard cues that my patient wanted to maintain her privacy and did not want to interact. I had witnessed the tail end of this interaction when I went to meet this patient.

In this disruptive incident, Sylvia was repeating the intrusive behavior that caused her difficulty at school. By behaving aggressively in my waiting room, she might have been expressing anger toward me. She might also have resented sharing me with the other woman, and might have felt competitive with her, particularly after I had previously criticized Sylvia's behavior. I wanted Sylvia to talk about feelings rather than act on them (as she had done in my waiting room). By addressing this issue, I hoped to help Sylvia, but I also wanted to try to ensure that this behavior did not repeat.

I recognized the fragility of my alliance with Sylvia, but given what was at stake for me and for my other patient, I felt that I had to confront her. In our next session I told Sylvia that I wanted people within my suite to be able to maintain their privacy. She seemed surprised, hurt, and became defensive. She accused me of caring about everyone but her. I think she could not tolerate my caring about anyone but her, and my concern about the other patient made Sylvia feel that I did not care about her at all. She denied that her behavior had been inappropriate or intrusive. It was possible that Sylvia did not read nonverbal signals from my other patient, who was not very assertive. But it was also possible that she had chosen to intentionally disregard these cues because she wanted interaction or because she wanted to provoke me.

Knowing that her father would side with her, Sylvia immediately told him that I had again criticized her. In the next session Sylvia reported to me that he thought that I was "out of line" and that I did not know how an office should be run. I asked whether Sylvia might have wanted her father to criticize me because I had criticized her. She denied that she would want him to be angry with me, but she acknowledged that she felt hurt and angry. Sylvia had been hurt when I questioned her flirtatious behavior, but the sting of that confrontation was softened by the fact that she knew I had only her welfare in mind. Now she felt that I put someone else's welfare above her own—she could no longer entertain the fantasy that she was my only priority.

This was a critical juncture in the treatment. Sylvia had introduced into our relationship and into my work space the very issues that we had been exploring at arm's length regarding her social interactions at school. She had done so in a manner in which I would have a personal stake in her behavior. I was no longer in the role of observer, but rather I was directly impacted.

At this point, Sylvia had to confront a painful conflict. She wanted to continue seeing herself as a very special person who was not being given a chance by her superficial peers. She also wanted to avoid a sense of responsibility for her social difficulties, but if she carried none of the fault, there would be nothing she could do to improve her experience at school. To make more friends, she would have to be more patient in developing social connections, more sensitive to the feelings of the other, and more able to tolerate rejection without reacting aggressively. But neither she nor her father wanted to acknowledge that she might have social problems. His negative reaction to my confrontation distracted from this work. We were talking about his objections instead of exploring why Sylvia approached my other patient, whether she noticed the cues this woman was giving to be left alone, and how Sylvia felt if she *had* picked up on the patient's attempt to limit their contact.

I did not know whether Sylvia, despite her loneliness, would be willing to try to attend to the feelings of others and prioritize their needs at least some of the time. Sylvia might have needed parental support to confront her tendency to be self-absorbed and to develop more capacity for mutuality. She would likely be unable to overcome her wishes for unconditional love and acceptance from peers while her father was confirming that these expectations were reasonable.

Up to this point, Sylvia's father had pursued no contact with me beyond a few calls to update me regarding his daughter's level of stress or medical status. Now, he phoned to register concern that I had upset Sylvia. He said it was inappropriate for me to criticize Sylvia and that she should be able to behave as she wished in my waiting room. Mr. F said that he would continue to support the treatment as long as Sylvia wanted it, but he felt that Sylvia was no longer benefiting and that, in fact, she seemed to be getting worse—she seemed angrier. Sylvia had gotten into a fight with him and with her mother and had "talked back." Previously, Sylvia tended to be compliant. She would sulk when she was angry, but she would not directly challenge her parents. He disapproved of this change. Mr. F did acknowledge, however, that Sylvia seemed less anxious, which I attributed to her developing ability to express anger.

In her conflicts with me, Sylvia had verbalized her anger, communicating directly and with specificity what I had done to offend her. Although she did not let go of her anger, she was more willing to converse about her feelings than I would have expected. I also suspected that Sylvia might have been exaggerating her anger because she did not want to concede that she could have been doing anything wrong. I acknowledged to Mr. F that it can be unpleasant and perhaps difficult to deal with Sylvia's anger but that she could benefit from expressing her feelings. I explained that she was making progress in the treatment.

Mr. F remained skeptical. I had underestimated the extent to which Sylvia would invite this intrusion and the aggressive way that he would step in. At this point, I needed to deal directly with his negative reactions to the treatment; my plan to work with Sylvia apart from her parents was no longer feasible. Based on the way in which Sylvia dealt with our conflict, I could see I had overestimated her readiness to operate independently from her father.

It had become clear that I would not be able to provide the kind of separate space for Sylvia that I had hoped, and I needed to renegotiate the boundaries of our work. I suggested to Mr. F that we meet to discuss his daughter's treatment, but he declined. After a few more sessions with Sylvia, Mr. F called to inform me that Sylvia had told him that she wanted to stop the therapy.

Mr. F did not want me to challenge his view of his daughter and the nature of her problems. It is not necessarily problematic for a therapist and a parent to have different perspectives, provided that there is a foundation of trust and mutual respect in their relationship. Such trust does not have to depend on contact between parent and therapist. Recognizing their daughter's need for her own treatment, parents may decide to support the therapy from the sidelines, through its inevitable ups and downs. To the extent that a young woman can operate independently of her parents, she also might be able to tolerate areas of conflict between her family and her therapist. An adolescent might know that she needs a different perspective. I was promoting critical self-reflection, which challenged the family tendency to blame others. It might have been threatening for Sylvia to take responsibility for her behavior and to venture down a path that was different from what her father would want for her. Had she been willing to tolerate my challenge and maintain a boundary around her treatment, she would have taken a step toward separating from him.

There were obvious differences between my perspective and that of her father, but I failed to anticipate the force of family-based opposition that was to develop. Had I been working with both of her parents, I might have been able to explore their reaction to Sylvia's emotional and social struggles and their reasons for resisting therapeutic change. I also might have been able to prevent the split that ultimately undermined my alliance with Sylvia.

By operating outside of the family domain, I was vulnerable to being seen as the problem (like the classmates who would not befriend Sylvia). When I undertook treatment of Sylvia independent of her parents, I might have been influenced by her father's inclination to overstate Sylvia's capacities. But even after the resistance had played out, I was still not sure whether a different approach might have yielded a different outcome. If I had pushed more in the beginning to include her parents in the treatment, or recommend parent guidance from another therapist who could work with their resistance while allowing Sylvia to have her own therapeutic relationship with me, the therapy might have gone further. But I am quite sure that they would have refused either of these options.

Sylvia's parents would likely maintain their denial until their daughter's problems began to impact on areas of functioning that they personally valued, such as her academic performance. Despite her emotional and social difficulties, Sylvia was getting good grades in high school, which her parents took as evidence that she did not have problems. I told her parents that I expected that Sylvia might have more difficulty when she went away to college, and they could no longer buffer the rejection and isolation she would likely experience—which might impact her academic functioning. She lacked the skills to develop the solid peer support that she would need to separate from her family. It was likely that only academic failure would provide incentive for her parents to recognize the severity of her problems and support psychotherapy.

Did the Treatment Fail?

After Sylvia left therapy, I asked myself whether the treatment had failed or more specifically what it meant that she left treatment prematurely (at least from my perspective). I felt that Sylvia had forced my hand, provoking confrontation she could or would not tolerate, possibly sabotaging her own therapy. The provocative nature of Sylvia's resistance might indicate that the treatment was too threatening—she might not have been ready to address her interpersonal impact, at least not without parental support. She might also have been overwhelmed by dependent longings in our relationship, which may have been more intense because of her limited contact with her mother. In that case, she might have pulled her father into her treatment to defuse our bond.

In my effort to work with Sylvia, I found myself in a bind. I knew that any confrontation could jeopardize the treatment, but to withhold my concerns about Sylvia's flirtatious behavior would have been negligent and possibly dangerous, especially because she did not seem to recognize the risk. I did not think that Sylvia had intended to provoke a confrontation around this issue, but she did use our confrontation to provoke her father to oppose me. I believe that Sylvia did intentionally provoke the second confrontation because she was angry with me, and I had no choice but to react. I could not sacrifice the comfort of my other patient to avoid a potentially damaging conflict with Sylvia. But perhaps my biggest problem was that I was constricted by Sylvia's parents, who refused to participate in the treatment or allow me to work autonomously with her.

Sylvia may not have been ready to engage in therapeutic work that would challenge her view of herself and her parents' view of her. Given her difficulty developing social relationships, it may have been more appropriate to start with family-based therapy or at least conjoint therapy with her father, had this been possible. Sylvia may have felt more comfortable and less conflicted if her parents had been involved, her attachment to me might have felt less regressive, and consequently she might have had less need to provoke critical reactions. But because Sylvia's own resistance was joined by that of her parents, it was more difficult to address. The seemingly premature termination likely reflected the limit of how far Sylvia and her family were able to progress therapeutically at that time.

The problems that developed over the course of the treatment could perhaps have been anticipated but not avoided. A patient's resistance can overwhelm a treatment. Although Sylvia never inflicted any physical self-injury, she might have been struggling with self-destructive impulses that caused her to place herself in danger with men and, perhaps, to sabotage a treatment that represented her best hope to learn how to make friends and build an attachment outside of her family.

Resistance is particularly complicated in work with adolescents, as their dependence on parents introduces more possible sources of opposition. Parents will influence an adolescent's experience of therapy, a daughter can provoke doubt or skepticism in her parents, and the family may find union in shared criticism of a therapist. Parents may be personally threatened by acknowledging problems in a daughter as well as her growing capacity for autonomy. They may feel competitive with their daughter's therapeutic attachment and a therapist's wish to emotionally nurture. Even when therapists work with the family, which is not always possible or appropriate, they may not be able to effectively address the various influences on an adolescent's treatment.

An outcome that looks like therapeutic failure may in fact reflect the limits of what an adolescent and her family can tolerate at a particular time. The decision to leave treatment may feel like a rejection of the therapist. But the adolescent may actually feel attached and might even be ending treatment because she or her parents cannot tolerate this attachment. Although the clinical work and opportunity for further therapeutic growth has been aborted, possibly in the service of protecting dysfunctional patterns within the family, the therapy might nonetheless have continuing influence. The adolescent will have gained experience that is different from what might be available within her family and she may become aware that there are other ways of relating. She may begin to question familiar self-defeating patterns, even if she is not ready to give them up. A short therapy that ends abruptly and with feelings of anger or dissatisfaction can still provide a sense of different possibilities that may be pursued at some later point, perhaps with a different therapist when the adolescent becomes more independent from parents and has developed more connections outside of her family.

Chapter 4

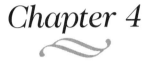

Challenging Resistance
and Sustaining Attachment

If therapists become too hesitant to confront resistance, they can feel as if they are walking on eggshells. Without intending to do so, they could wind up avoiding conflict, possibly repeating the young woman's experience with parents who did not confront problems. The patient may feel accepted, but she may also suspect that the therapist is not being entirely genuine. Is there something so wrong with her that the therapist cannot address it? Does the therapist think that she is too fragile? Moreover, if she is not responsible, at least to some extent, for the problems in her life, then she has less leverage to effect change. Therefore, while confrontation can challenge and perhaps even threaten the therapeutic relationship, it can also build trust that the patient and therapist can deal with difficult things together—that the therapist is willing to take the risk of offering honest feedback. The ability to effectively confront a patient reflects, at least in part, the existence of a healthy, resilient therapeutic relationship, and the experience of dealing with conflict may, in turn, further deepen this relationship. Thus, rather than shying away from confrontation altogether, therapists might instead proceed in a manner that is mindful of the adaptive functions of resistance, the patient's vulnerabilities, the state of the therapeutic relationship, as well as the emotional impact of any critical feedback they might offer.

When therapists confront resistance, there is always risk that they could threaten the patient's coping mechanisms as well as her trust and comfort in the treatment relationship. A young woman who is unprepared to change may fear that she is disappointing the therapist by holding on to patterns that have been identified as dysfunctional. She may become hesitant to expose aspects of attachments that she knows to be self-defeating. If she feels too injured by the therapist, she may become less open to clinical exploration, and the scope of the treatment may become more limited.

Given the potential risk to the therapeutic relationship, therapists may feel uncertain about whether or when they should confront problematic patterns. Such was the case in my work with Beth. In the initial months of treatment, I had taken a consistently supportive tact, sympathizing with her past experience with an abusing parent. In an attempt to address her baseless sense of responsibility for her father's sexually violating behavior when she was a vulnerable child, I had helped Beth to see herself as a victim. However, as our focus shifted to her current life, my view of Beth broadened. I became concerned about Beth's role in what I was coming to regard as a pattern of job failures. She wanted me to empathize with her current problems at work, to validate her sense of being victimized (as I had in relation to her father), and to support her efforts to set limits with her boss.

But I was less sympathetic with her job-related complaints than Beth wanted and expected me to be. Rather than perceiving her as a victim of an exploitative boss, I felt that Beth might be inappropriately challenging her boss's authority. I actually thought she should probably work harder to meet his expectations. Conflict with former bosses had already cost her several jobs, and I could see that her current situation was also deteriorating. Perhaps it was not that her boss was exploitative, like her father, but that her anger toward her father caused her to provoke her boss in a manner that elicited a familiar controlling response. By failing to accept his authority, she might have been shaping his behavior to be more like that of her dominating father. I thought that her efforts to be "self-protective" had a defiant quality in the context of a boss–employee relationship, and I was concerned that she would get fired again.

Yet, I recognized that if I failed to provide an empathic outlet for her distress, Beth might be less able to tolerate the job stress, and she could become more provocative or less able to cope at work. If I suggested that I did not think that her boss's demands were as unreasonable as she believed, she might feel betrayed, isolated again with no protective caregiver to whom she could turn. But at the same time I did not want her to lose her job, and so become more dependent on her family. In addition to being a victim in relation to her father, Beth could also be aggressive—like him. She had pressured me to support her negative view of her boss, for example.

Beth was not seeking therapeutic confrontation, but that did not mean that she could not tolerate it and benefit from it. There would be risks involved in introducing challenge, particularly because she had grown accustomed to a therapeutic response that she experienced as supportive—early in the treatment, I had been inclined to encourage her to *not* blame herself for things that had been beyond her control (like her father's abuse) and I tended to validate her feelings and viewpoint. These were reasons to be particularly cautious in shifting my stance with Beth. But therapists should always consider the possible impact of confrontation on the patient's experience of the therapeutic relationship. Therapists need to remain aware of the patient's response to the confrontation, particularly the possible detrimental impact of challenging a defense that has had adaptive value. A patient might be destabilized or antagonized. Because therapists cannot always anticipate the effect of confrontation, they must be prepared to back down—not necessarily to reverse their position but rather reduce pressure toward change. They must also remain alert for delayed, displaced, or disguised negative reactions that, if not addressed, could undermine the therapeutic alliance.

A young woman's reaction to challenge is influenced by the extent to which she continues to rely on resistance to fend off difficult feelings, to maintain a sense or herself, and to remain in connection with her family. It will also reflect the solidity of her relationship with the therapist, specifically whether she is able to sustain her attachment in the face of challenge. To assess a patient's readiness to tolerate confrontation, therapists might consider emotional and interpersonal capacities including the following:

- Is the young woman's emotional stability dependent on maintaining a particular view of herself and her relationships, which could be threatened by a challenge from the therapist?
- Are dysfunctional patterns rigidly rooted in her family? If she challenges her parents' view of her and of themselves, does she risk rejection?
- In therapeutic interaction or social relationships, does she resist taking on new perspectives and trying out new ways of relating?
- Can she manage anxiety and painful feelings?
- Can she tolerate disapproval or critical feedback, or would her ability to maintain self-esteem be threatened?
- Would her attachment to the therapist be jeopardized by disapproval, criticism, or conflict?

A patient may feel hurt or angry in response to confrontation even if she is able to deal with the challenge. In fact, her very ability to express anger, disagreement, or opposition could suggest that she is able to engage in conflict. Conversely, the absence of negative reaction does not mean that the patient is making productive use of the challenge. To protect the treatment, therapists must remain particularly attuned to reactions that are not verbalized. A patient may not trust the therapist with her negative responses. Instead of voicing feelings of anger or betrayal, she might pull back emotionally. If therapists fail to notice this shift and its relationship to the confrontation, they may be unable to restore trust and their emotional connection.

Providing a Protected Holding Space

Slochower (2005) highlights the value of therapeutic work that refrains from imposing the therapist's perspective. "We may be slower to recognize how clinical movement is sometimes effected not by our capacity to make meaning, but by our ability to create an emotional space within which inner experience can be articulated rather than challenged" (2005, p. 31). Vulnerable patients may need to be free to hold on to their own experience before they are ready to deal with a conflicting or even a merely different or separate viewpoint. In the face of this clinical need, therapists might try to provide what Holmes described as "nonintrusive attention" (1996, p. 125) or Slochower (2005) described as a "protective holding space" that can "crucially support the expression and exploration of heretofore dissociated or denied aspects of affective life" (p. 33). Within this environment, a young woman might become able to more fully and safely experience, accept, and integrate threatening feelings.

To create this supportive experience, the therapist needs to try to attune to the patient's emotional state, "to remain evenly and consistently present, intact and available" (p. 35). Any challenge or failure to attune could disrupt the feeling of connection. Consequently, input that reflects the therapist's opinion or perspective can feel "highly emotionally disjunctive, that is, 'out of sync' with a patient's affective state" (Slochower, 2005, p. 33). According to Slochower (2005), "holding" "always involves the analyst's struggle to establish a contained emotional space within which a range of difficult experiences can be experienced and expressed" (p. 34).

Slochower (2005) acknowledges, however, that holding is an "*illusion* of analytic reliability and attunement" (p. 34; italics added). "The holding space is not established by the analyst alone; patients unconsciously participate in sustaining the holding experience by excluding aspects of the analyst's presence that threaten to disrupt it. In this sense the holding experience requires the patient's implicit participation" (p. 37). If the patient seizes upon the inevitable moments when the therapist misses the mark emotionally, she makes it impossible to create a holding experience. Slochower distinguishes the "tacit negotiations" that allow a therapist and patient to create an illusion of attunement from the "very explicit negotiations" (p. 37) that are required by more mutual interaction.

When working with patients who are vulnerable in the way that Slochower described, therapists must prioritize efforts to empathize and attune over their inclination to offer their own perspective, even if their intent is to provide support. In my work with Sonya, I failed to recognize the potentially disruptive impact of shifting from an empathic stance to an attempt at problem solving. Although I did not intend to challenge Sonya, my input proved to be an intrusion, which at least temporarily disrupted our connection and her sense of emotional safety. I made this misstep with full awareness that Sonya was vulnerable. As a freshman who had left her single mother to attend college, Sonya had been unable to create a comfortable niche at school. She confided that I was her only source of emotional support—actually, I was the only person with whom she talked more than superficially. She needed therapy to provide a haven from the agitation she experienced in her daily life.

Sonya was deeply attached to a mother who was very limited in her ability to provide support. Ms. T seemed to be even more emotionally vulnerable than her daughter. She had never married, she earned little money, and she clung to physically abusive, alcoholic men, on whom she depended for financial support. Sonya was relieved to move away from these men, but she seemed unable to cope with the separation from her mother.

Her closest tie outside of her mother in high school was with a best girlfriend. Each served as the other's primary social connection, and it seemed natural to Sonya when their relationship became a bit sexual. But after a few months, her friend seemed to panic about their sexual contact. Rather than just returning to their formerly platonic relationship, she rejected Sonya altogether and began to spend all her time with a new boyfriend. Sonya was devastated both by the rejection and the loss, and she subsequently kept largely to herself at school.

By college, she had not learned how to make friends or soothe herself, other than by smoking marijuana. She was lonely and felt that she belonged only when sharing pot. Sonya struggled to develop a solid connection to me. She was willing to use me for support, but she did not seem to be looking to develop an emotional attachment. I functioned mostly as a sounding board. Sonya felt guilty about getting help that was unavailable to her mother. By depending on me, she felt that she was being disloyal. Yet, despite the limitations she imposed on the treatment, Sonya was probably more attached to me than to anyone other than her high school girlfriend and her mother.

In therapy, Sonya talked mostly about her struggle to manage her part-time job in addition to the demands of school. She was becoming increasingly exhausted and depleted. I felt that she might have taken on too much. As I listened to her frenetic attempt to keep up, my empathy did not feel sufficient. I did not seem to be helping her manage better, and she had no other means to find even temporary relief, other than smoking pot. For several months, I stuck with this emotionally supportive position, but as I saw her stress mount, I thought I might try to help a bit more actively. I suggested that Sonya try to pace herself, and I proposed that we might work together, right then, to figure out ways that she could lighten her load. I had hoped to help Sonya lower her stress—I did not think I was posing a challenge. But I immediately saw that she felt threatened. She became agitated. She said she had told me too much and insisted that she couldn't make more changes now. She complained that she couldn't talk about it any more and then fell silent.

I was impressed that Sonya was able to verbalize her negative reaction as much as she did. As soon as I saw her distress, I immediately pulled back, retracting my suggestion. By making a shift from empathizing with her feelings to offering concrete suggestions, I had implied that she could exercise some control over the demands in her life. I had inadvertently imposed pressure to change—to find a way to manage better. Moreover, when I focused on the multiple sources of stress in her life, she might have felt that I was implying that her mother was a burden. For this reason, she could have reasonably feared that I was challenging her attachment to her mother, which was integral to Sonya's sense of self.

Immediately shifting back to my former supportive stance, I told Sonya that I understood that she was just too busy now, and I realized there might be nothing she could do about it. This shift in my thinking was genuine, as I had realized that Sonya was not yet able to slow down. She could not see that she might have the power to make any change and could not even imagine that life could be more manageable. I explained that I did not mean to impose pressure, that I recognized that her responsibilities were just overwhelming, and that I was glad she had been able to share with me her feelings of stress and her reaction to my feedback. Although I had not expected my intervention to be challenging, I had been aware that I was changing gears when I made the suggestion, and I had remained attuned to the possible impact on Sonya.

Sonya's sense of self revolved around the experience of being overwhelmed. I had thought she needed help regulating her level of activity and setting priorities, particularly because her mother had never provided such guidance. But I had underestimated the extent to which Sonya might have needed the chaos to avoid feeling her feelings and to maintain a connection with her mother and her childhood experience. When I suggested that she could exercise some control over the pace of her life, I was threatening the way that she organized her sense of herself and the way that she managed feelings. Had I persisted, Sonya might have had to retreat to a position of paranoid distrust so as to fend off my influence. I needed to return to my initial commitment to sit with her experience.

If Sonya became more emotionally stable from her therapeutic work, she might feel too different and separate from her mother—which might threaten their bond. I further suspected that if she began to feel too attached to me, she might flee out of loyalty to her mother. I had to accept Sonya's limitations and the value of providing an attachment that did not push beyond the boundary she had established.

I could also help Sonya even if I did not get her to take action to reduce her stress. By listening and empathizing, I could be present with Sonya with her stress, and I could provide a supportive connection outside of her mother. I could also notice moments of calm in our interaction, and by making Sonya aware of them, I might help her to recognize her capacity to feel a wider range of feelings. Sonya might gradually realize that she would not be empty if her life were less frenetic. I was also able to engage other parts of her personality, expressing appreciation for the way she loved and cared for abandoned animals or the funky creativity of her dress, which could help to expand her sense of self.

As I engaged with Sonya around these idiosyncratic aspects of her personality, I was also more able to attach to her. It had not been easy for me to connect with her because she presented so little feeling, maintained distance in our interactions, and could be unsettled by any imposition of my own views or personality. Her clothes, which revealed a more artistic bent that was not otherwise evident in our interaction, provided an avenue for not only helping Sonya to connect with different parts of herself but also for me to connect with her. It is not possible to attach to every patient, but the failure to do so can limit the treatment. Therefore, in the service of trying to connect, therapists need to actively look for what can spark their interest, what they can relate to, what is intriguingly different, and what they are touched by. In this way, they can work to build a bond despite interpersonal differences and the patient's own resistance.

I was providing new experience for Sonya that did not threaten her sense of self—a connection that did not revolve around shared chaos. My ability to remain calm in the face of Sonya's distress modeled a departure from Sonya's tendency to be consumed by her mother's emotional turmoil. I allowed for an experience of separation within the context of a relationship—I could be in a different state than Sonya and yet we could be connected. If applied to her relationship with her mother, she might feel that she could be okay even if her mother is not. This experience might enable her to maintain stability while feeling their connection. As Sonya develops new ways of seeing herself, awareness of calmer feelings, and the ability to feel bonded with her mother even when she is in a different state, she could be less threatened by the prospect of letting go of her frenetic level of activity.

Challenge Can Introduce a Fuller Range of Emotional Expression

A young woman who has more capacity to deal with feelings than Sonya might feel constrained by the type of holding environment that Sonya so desperately needed. The safety afforded by consistent empathic effort, which allowed Sonya to express a wider range of feelings, could limit or constrict emotional and relational potential with a patient who can deal with different viewpoints. Rather than relying upon "tacit negotiation" to maintain an illusion that the therapist is consistently tuned into her emotional experience, the patient might benefit from the opportunity to negotiate overtly and directly, exchange different viewpoints, and deal with conflict. New emotional experience might then emerge not from a haven that is safe from intrusion, but rather from interaction that invites discourse, challenge, feedback, and open expression of positive and negative reactions.

When she entered psychotherapy, Patricia was attached to a

view of herself as a caregiver. She did not care for her own health, however—she was obese and didn't invest the time to eat well or exercise. At a young age Patricia had married a successful businessman and was committed to caring for her husband and her widowed mother, disabled by a stroke, who lived with them. She valued selflessness and was reluctant to set limits with her husband or mother. She sacrificed her own needs to care for them, and they accepted whatever she offered without regard for the toll on her. With the addition of a new baby to the family, Patricia was overwhelmed. She became so depleted that she felt it necessary to seek therapy. She wanted help coping with the stress, but she was not willing to cut back on what she would provide her family.

Patricia was stressed not just by demands imposed by family members, but how they made her feel about herself. Her mother remained relentlessly critical and disapproving even in the face of Patricia's best efforts to please. Despite Patricia's painstaking care, her mother continued to smoke, drink, and overeat. Patricia denied feeling angry about any of these provocations. She desperately wanted to secure approval from her mother, who had never told Patricia that she loved her. If Patricia expressed frustration with her mother, she would be plagued by guilt and passive suicidal wishes. Then she would try to compensate for her negative reaction by making more sacrifices.

I asked Patricia if she were angry, despite her belief that she had no reason to be. With this question, I was challenging her defensive stance, which was based on a denial of anger. I felt she might be able to deal with this challenge because she had already told me many things about her mother that she knew had made me angry toward her mother. Nonetheless, I was not surprised when Patricia denied feeling angry. Unlike Sonya, she did not seem to be threatened by my challenge. Rather than becoming disorganized, panicked, or withdrawn, Patricia seemed enlivened. She may not have been ready to give up the defense, but she seemed to be using my question to begin to entertain a different perspective on her relationship with her mother.

Yet, I stopped short of challenging her caregiving role. Patricia was ambivalent about treatment, and her decision to seek help itself represented a departure—she had begun to consider her needs. I did not want to push her to go too far, too fast, and I wanted to respect what she felt she needed from treatment, which was help coping with stress. Therefore, I would try to enable her to better care for herself within the constraints of her caregiving role. I wanted to offer my emotional support and provide a relationship for Patricia that was centered on her needs.

Several months into the treatment, Patricia arrived for her session in extreme distress. I suspected that with the strain of suppressed anger, her mother's relentless demands had become overwhelming, particularly when piled on the demands of caring for a new baby. Patricia felt that she could not cope, she felt hopeless and helpless, and she was preoccupied with suicidal thoughts, though she had no plan or intent to act.

I told Patricia that I thought her mother was becoming unmanageable, and I worried that as a result, she, Patricia, might become unable to maintain her own emotional stability. I expressed my concern that she would take self-destructive action or, more likely, that the pressure could compromise her emotional and physical health. Patricia binged on junk food when she was stressed, and I could see that she was gaining weight at an alarming rate. She admitted to feeling desperately distressed, but she refused my recommendation to consider a brief inpatient stay, or to find some other way to get a break from her family that would allow her to stabilize emotionally.

When Patricia remained unable to find respite, I suggested that she might consider helping her mother move to an assisted living situation. In this way, she could use her financial resources to get care for mother without depleting herself. Patricia was appalled by my suggestion. She said that she was responsible for her mother and would never abandon her. If I could even consider the possibility that she send her mother away, then I did not know her at all. I noticed her growing more distant, and she explained that she was shutting down, she couldn't help it. She refused to talk further about her reactions to my suggestion. I feared that my effort to advocate for her had posed too great a challenge to her identity as caregiver. She wanted to believe that she must do all that she was doing. I was suggesting that she had more control and ability to care for herself than she could accept.

In the next session Patricia told me that she had thought she might not return and, now that she was here, she was not sure she should have come. She was angry, and she had decided to come to let me know it. I considered backing down, particularly as I feared she could quit treatment. However, I recognized that her ability to get angry with me was a huge step forward. If I backed down, I risked communicating that I could not tolerate her anger. I did not push the idea of assisted living any further, but I also did not apologize for suggesting it. She complained that it was inappropriate for me to tell her what to do with her mother and asserted that I was pressuring her to do something that was not right for her. By exposing her frustration and distress, Patricia had stimulated me to advocate for her, but she was not yet ready to take self-protective action.

Unlike Sonya, who became so threatened that she could barely continue talking to me, Patricia got angry. So I held my ground. I told Patricia I still thought it might be better both for herself and for her mother if she considered an assisted living option, but I respected that she had a different viewpoint. I told her that I did not want to pressure her to do what I was suggesting, and I felt it was okay to differ even on such an important issue. Patricia had never before openly addressed conflict in a caregiving relationship. She always felt that she must do what her mother wanted, and she was never permitted to disagree. Based on her past experience, Patricia expected that she would either have to comply with my recommendation, which was out of the question given her sense of obligation to her mother, or leave me.

I wanted to deal with our conflict. She had broken new ground by verbalizing her anger and showing angry affect. Although I did not reverse my position, I accepted responsibility for making her angry. I explained that it was possible to stay connected while maintaining our different viewpoints and that I did not feel less invested in her because she rejected my suggestion. She was surprised that her anger toward me did not make her feel guilty.

Over the weeks that followed, Patricia began to comment, at heated moments, that she "hated" her mother, and she noticed that she did not feel suicidal. And she no longer cried when she expressed negative feelings. She had become more comfortable with her anger partly because she had gotten angry with me, and we had continued to be close.

Several weeks later, Patricia told me that she was considering the possibility of placing her mother in an assisted care facility. She had recognized the toll her mother's presence was taking not only her, but on her marriage. She and her husband had been growing more distant. Patricia recognized that she might be feeling less tolerant of her husband's demanding, unappreciative attitude toward her, but she also thought that the stress introduced by her mother might be playing a role. It was possible that Patricia had been dealing with so much suppressed anger that she could think of assisted living only as a punishment for her mother. Now that she was more able to accept her anger, she was also more able to see the possible benefits for herself and her mother. This perspective represented a departure from her defensive stance, in which she tried to deny anger and atone for her negative reactions through self-sacrifice.

If the patient does not accept the therapist's perspective or chooses not to implement a particular recommendation, then she and the therapist must live with some tension in their relationship. The therapy might move on to address other issues, with disagreement lingering but relegated to the background. The challenge may fade from immediate attention, possibly to be reintroduced as the problem resurfaces or the patient becomes ready to deal with the challenge. As they approach confrontation, therapists must accept patients' freedom to reject their input. The patient also must struggle to tolerate her differences from the therapist and the fact that her therapist disagrees with her choice. Further, she must face her responsibility for what change she does or does not choose to implement.

Therapeutic Challenge May Threaten a Patient's Autonomy

As a patient begins to assert autonomy, she might make choices that defy or disappoint the therapist. Like parents, therapists may need to stand by while an adolescent experiments, explores, struggles, and flounders as she begins to individuate and find her niche in the world. In this context, challenge could be experienced by the patient as a threat to her autonomy. When therapists intervene, even in an attempt to protect treatment gains or the patient's well-being, they may communicate a lack of confidence in her choices. Even as an adolescent acts defiantly, she may want to share her experience, and she may need the therapist to trust that she can manage independently.

Throughout the first year of Karla's treatment, we experienced no conflict, nor had I felt any inclination to challenge her. I recognized that our relationship represented Karla's only significant tie outside of her family, and I was eager to nurture her attachment. Karla had experienced very minimal emotional support from her family. Her mother mocked her attempts to make friends or join in school activities. She had convinced Karla that people could not be trusted and would inevitably take advantage of her. Although she was almost thirty years old, Karla had never had a boyfriend or a close girlfriend. She had learned to be quite self-sufficient and seemed content pursuing interests on her own. Karla resented her mother's interference in her life, but she remained devoted. As disappointing as her family was, Karla believed that this was the best she could expect in any relationship.

Karla was so eager to be accepted that she was reluctant to set self-protective limits or assert her needs. Consequently, she was often exploited, just as her mother had warned. Supposed friends would borrow money that they would fail to repay. If they asked for another loan, Karla would not refuse them for fear that she would be rejected. Karla had no experience getting her needs met in relationships, and she did not know how to choose or cultivate mutually supportive friendships.

Psychotherapy presented an opportunity to focus on her emotional experience, but she clearly did not trust me. In sessions, she spoke in the most general terms, revealing little about her daily life or her feelings. To respect her boundaries, I avoided probing questions. I wanted to get to know Karla better, but it seemed more important to give her room to approach treatment on her own terms. Karla's seemed fearful that, like her mother, I would criticize her and undermine her confidence that she could do what she wanted. She tried to limit her disclosure to protect her freedom to make her own choices.

Karla began to pursue an interest in travel, which seemed to reflect increasing willingness to invest in herself. But she maintained her privacy around these plans as well, and she seemed relieved that I would just listen attentively. Within these constraints, I had little opportunity to show that I could support her choices.

Nonetheless, she seemed to be using therapy to develop her life. Due to her travels, she began to miss some therapy sessions, but her absences seemed driven by schedule conflicts arising from her growing independence rather than by resistance. At first, it appeared that her travel would be a solitary pursuit, like her other hobbies had been. But when Karla returned from one of her trips, she informed me that she had met a man, Dan, whom she really liked. She had already planned an extended return visit and would stay at Dan's house.

By becoming involved with Dan, she was taking a huge leap from the world of her apartment, her cats, and her family. She seemed to me to be moving forward quickly, given that she had had so little prior dating experience. From my perspective, she barely knew Dan. But I also recognized that Karla was trying to build new relationships and experience and to trust someone outside of her family. Moreover, despite her fear that I would question her judgment, she told me of her plan, which represented a departure from her prior, more guarded, stance with me.

I recognized that Karla needed to take risks. She was launching into the exploration that she did not have the opportunity to pursue in adolescence. She had not learned how to assert her needs, to negotiate, to set self-protective limits, to deal with sex, or to handle rejection. Now, in adulthood, the stakes of experimentation were higher. I was concerned that impulsive action might undermine the stability she had achieved, but if she did not take some chances in new relationships, Karla would not be able to develop. To help with this process, I had been recommending that she join one of my psychotherapy groups where she could make connections with, and gain exposure to, the life experience of other young women. But the idea of beginning to make social connections through therapy did not appeal to her.

Although I felt concerned about her rush to be with Dan, I recognized that her interest in this relationship was probably an outgrowth of our work. She did not allow herself to get her emotional needs met in therapy, but the process did stimulate her interest in developing other relationships. As she became more aware of her needs, she began to long for a romantic relationship. Yet she was not experienced at evaluating a potential partner; she had not had the opportunity to develop a sense of what might signal potential problems, nor did she really know what to look for in a relationship. I could encourage Karla to talk about her feelings and experience with Dan, and help her to anticipate pitfalls, but I could not protect her.

I felt too much responsibility as the only person who knew of Karla's plans with Dan. I wanted to be as protective as possible without jeopardizing her trust or comfort with me. If familiar patterns were to play out here, she might pick up on my concern and retreat to a position of self-doubt, in which she resents but submits to my authority, as she did with her mother, and misses out on yet another opportunity because of the skepticism and fears of a caregiver. If she felt that I was trying to undermine her plan in any way, she might shore up her defenses more aggressively against my influence and proceed to go through the motions of therapy in the absence of genuine emotional engagement.

I genuinely wanted to support her relationship with Dan, but I also recognized that I did not have the leverage to hold her back, even if I had wanted to. I did not hide my concerns, but I was measured in expressing them. I acknowledged that Karla was taking a big leap, and I asked whether she had thought about pacing the relationship, but I emphasized that I was not trying to influence her decision to be with Dan. In fact, I was not hoping to convince her of anything, except to think about her options as broadly as possible.

I also wanted to give her room to talk about her concerns regarding Dan without fear that I would use them as ammunition against the relationship. Trying to help her anticipate potential pressures, I asked whether she had thought about sex. I would not judge any desire she might have, but given that she could not refuse a friend's request for money, I thought she might have difficulty setting limits with Dan. It turned out that Karla had thought about this area and explained that she would leave Dan and go to a hotel if she became uncomfortable. She further reassured me that she could fly home early if she wanted. I was beginning to have more confidence that she could act self-protectively, which I tried to communicate to Karla.

Rather than confronting dangers or pressing her to change her plans, I wanted to understand Karla's experience of Dan. I wanted to know what he was like, what she enjoyed about him, and what she hoped to get from their relationship. She explained that Dan did things for her, which made daily life feel less burdensome. He had helped her with her travel arrangements, for example. She had never before experienced support of this kind, and she wanted to trust him and incorporate him into her life. I suggested that she might be experiencing a greater sense of need now that she had someone in her life who might respond. With this type of gratification seemingly possible, it would feel bleak to return to the routine of self-sufficiency. Karla cried. She said that before meeting Dan, she had been struggling to rearrange her furniture and had had no one to turn to for help.

I wanted to offer Karla the opportunity to consider both the positive and negative aspects of the relationship, without fear that I would judge her. She admitted that she feared being hurt, as she has been in the past, but more than this she feared that she could lose this opportunity and live her life alone. Had I challenged her more vigorously, I would have risked pushing her into a defensive position, in which she would have represented only one side of her feelings: the hope and belief that she had found love. Karla would have defended her decision more adamantly and might not have acknowledged her fears.

As we talked about her relationship with Dan, I became more aware of the black-and-white nature of Karla's thinking. She believed that she must stay in Dan's apartment to establish a relationship, and that he would make her life fulfilling. However, she was beginning to use therapy to consider their relationship in a more complex way. She began to recognize that she might not be able to prevent potential disappointment even if she did everything that Dan wanted, and more generally that she could not control the course of a relationship as much as she might want.

Thinking about the possibility of being loved, Karla reflected on all that her parents failed to provide. I hoped that exploring the influence of her family experience might defuse the pressure to latch onto Dan as a panacea for her longstanding sense of deprivation. Karla knew that I cared about her, but our relationship did not provide the companionship that she craved. Moreover, our work was difficult and uncomfortable, lacking in the immediate gratification that she could get from a boyfriend. Karla longed for someone to go out with her and take care of her. I recognized that the hopes she attached to Dan could overwhelm her tenuous connection to me and that she might, at some point, leave me to be with him. Increasingly, the reflective nature of our work seemed to conflict with pressure from Dan and her own desperation to act.

A therapist could reasonably confront Karla's rush to Dan as a form of acting out, a flight from, or defense against, her clinical work. However, in making this challenge, the therapist might be overlooking the potentially progressive aspects of the relationship. By voicing a more skeptical position, I risked being experienced like Karla's mother. It was difficult to evaluate at this point what her relationship with Dan meant for Karla's development. But I knew that it was a sensitive issue. If I tried to exert too much control, I could damage our relationship. I did not want to tell her what to do, even how to pace her involvement with Dan. My goal was to help Karla explore her hopes and doubts, not impose my own.

Following her visit with Dan, which did not present any of the immediate dangers I had anticipated, their relationship began to move forward with greater speed. Karla continued to share with me her experience and her plans, but she became more detached from her feelings and from me, and more caught up in Dan. Even with the opportunity to consider and express her feelings, she did not slow her pace or reflect on her experience or decisions. In fact, soon after her visit, she announced that she would be leaving her job and her treatment, moving in with Dan in another state, and starting a landscaping business with him.

Although I understood how she could be captivated by Dan's attention and affection, I was frustrated and angered by the apparent ease with which she could let go of our connection and dismiss the value of our work and relationship as well as the life she had built. She had become determined to center her life on Dan, and she was quite willing to dismiss me. Dan had become everything that she needed, and I had become expendable. I continued to worry about Karla being exploited by Dan, but based on my experience with Karla, I also came to recognize that she might be using Dan too. She looked to Dan to fill the emptiness in her life, to escape from the boredom and frustration, and to take care of her. Dan's potential to exploit likely far exceeded that of Karla, but I suspected that she also brought some self-serving motives to the relationship.

There was certainly an argument to be made for trying to intervene in Karla's impulsive pursuit of Dan. Karla would lose her job, her home, her treatment, and she could be emotionally and financially devastated if she joined with Dan and their relationship and/or their business venture were to implode—a likely outcome from my vantage point. But if I challenged her, I risked damaging our relationship, possibly irreparably. Karla might experience me as possessive, like her mother. I had expected that Karla might leave treatment to be with Dan, and now that she seemed on the verge of separating from me, I wanted her to continue to feel our connection. I hoped that if she did leave, she might keep in touch or possibly resume therapy at some point, perhaps with me on the phone or with a new therapist. I did not want her to feel humiliated if she and Dan broke up or think that I might feel vindicated. I would remain available not because I expected or hoped that the relationship would fail (although I was skeptical), but because I wanted her to be able to follow her passion and still know that I was there for her if she needed me.

When a patient expresses anger and dissatisfaction with treatment, or when, like Karla, she pushes ahead with choices that fly in the face of treatment goals, therapists might feel that they have failed. At such difficult junctures, there is reason to be concerned about the patient and the treatment, but this type of challenge to the therapist might in fact reflect the patient's effort to assert her independence. The treatment relationship can survive conflict and disappointment, and it can be altered in ways that allow for greater separation in the context of connection. A young woman may need to reject therapeutic influence or even leave therapy to assert that she is able to live life on her own terms. If she were to feel so dependent on the therapist that she could not move away from treatment, then she could not feel fully separate and autonomous.

Chapter 5

~~~

The Going Gets Tough
When the Patient Gets Angry

*A*ttachment is no less meaningful or therapeutically valuable when it incorporates anger—even persistent, intense anger. A young woman may turn to conflict or defiance to create distance when she feels too dependent or vulnerable, not to detach from the therapist, but to protect her attachment. If she gets angry, she may be asserting herself and engaging more genuinely with the therapist, perhaps exploring new interpersonal territory. She may also use the therapeutic relationship to contain rage or self-loathing. By directing these feelings toward the therapist, she may protect against self-destructive behavior or preoccupation.

Especially when it represents a departure from more collaborative or harmonious interaction, anger and conflict can destabilize a therapeutic relationship. The patient might be frightened when expressing anger toward her therapist, expecting that it will trigger retaliation or abandonment, jeopardizing her primary emotional support. Her anger may threaten an idealization that has provided her with comfort and security. The therapeutic relationship may feel endangered. Even a mild, appropriately moderated annoyed or frustrated response from a therapist can feel like rejection. And therapists can in fact be injured and worn down, particularly by persistent anger or hostility. Under the weight of preponderant and seemingly unreasonable criticism, therapists may come to question their value to the patient. If they pull back emotionally or even consider ending the treatment, they may deprive the patient of a stable base of attachment at a time of heightened need. Therefore, as anger and conflict are introduced into the therapeutic relationship, there is potential for emotional and interpersonal growth and also risk of rupture.

As a therapist in a partial hospital program, I worked with patients who tended to avoid emotional dependence and to deal with feelings through self-destructive behavior. Sophia had a long history of depression, anorexia, and self-injury, and she came to the program following an extended hospitalization for a life-threatening suicide attempt. Inpatient treatment did little to contain her destructive impulses, in fact she made a second suicide attempt while in the hospital. I was Sophia's individual therapist within the partial program, but I was also part of a treatment team. With the support of my colleagues and the opportunity to manage risk collaboratively, I had the freedom to focus on developing my relationship with Sophia, and so I could more comfortably open myself to attach to her. Despite her disparaging attitude toward treatment, Sophia connected to me.

But her growing attachment, which I welcomed, quickly triggered an angry backlash from Sophia and provocative efforts to push me away. She suddenly and unexpectedly became cold and hostile. She remained unmoved by my attempts to understand her anger, empathize with her frustration, or reestablish a feeling of connection. She complained about me to other patients, who also began to target me with their anger. Even within my treatment team, I felt isolated and began to resent Sophia.

What happened to our attachment? Why did Sophia become so angry with me? How could I remain emotionally available and therapeutically helpful when I was angry at the way that she was treating me? There are dangers associated with attachment, particularly with patients such as Sophia who are fearful of emotional connection. Sophia made me doubt the value of the therapy I was providing, and her open expression of anger toward me within the program provoked distrust among other patients as well.

I was caught between the need to protect myself from Sophia's anger and a wish to protect Sophia from feeling rejected by my reaction to her anger. Although I could be hurt by Sophia, I was more concerned that she would turn her anger on herself. I also feared that her anger could overwhelm my ability to stay engaged therapeutically with her. I believe that the anger that Sophia expressed in treatment was only the tip of the iceberg. Her suppressed rage and potential for self-destructive behavior were extreme, but many patients will, like Sophia, direct negative reactions toward their therapists that do not necessarily reflect any thoughtful evaluation of the treatment. Later in the chapter, I describe the struggle that unfolded between us and my own struggle to deal therapeutically with the impact of her criticism and dissatisfaction.

Anger toward Mother

First, I take a step back to look at the connection between self-destructive behavior and difficulty expressing anger among young women, and more specifically, their tendency to turn anger inward, creating vulnerability to depression and self-defeating acting out. The bond between mothers and daughters can inhibit an adolescent's need to assert differences from her mother, triggering anger along with a need to suppress her anger. This deep empathic connection can make it difficult for the daughter to directly confront her mother with her resentment and frustration. Her anger, along with her press for self-determination, may be expressed in the form of rebellion, which may be self-defeating or even self-destructive. If a mother imposes pressure on her daughter to express affection or to resurrect the closeness more appropriate to childhood, she risks provoking more anger as the adolescent struggles to reinforce the boundary she has been trying to establish.

Because of her gender-based identification, a young woman has a special investment in her mother's choices, including those that do not directly impact on the mother's role as parent. The daughter may feel that her life is tied to her mother's life; she may understand that she could, intentionally or not, wind up making similar choices. A mother's self-defeating choices can thereby constrict her daughter's sense of self and possibility. A young woman may simultaneously feel inspired and pressured to equal her mother's achievements. She may also feel personally threatened and therefore angered by her mother's failures, which may seem to shape her own destiny.

A patient may bring anger into the treatment that she has been unable to express directly to her mother. It is often easier to talk about this anger with a therapist than express it within the family. There is less at stake in the treatment relationship and less concern about the therapist's potential vulnerability, at least relative to that of her mother, which can be liberating. At the same time, a therapist's emotionally nurturing role can elicit a sense of familial attachment, evoking familiar conflict. By verbalizing negative feelings that she may suppress in relation to her mother, an adolescent can potentially take a step toward dealing with anger in a caregiving relationship and away from directing it toward herself. The role of therapists may be similar to that of the parent in that therapists may need to absorb an adolescent's anger in the service of maintaining a stable attachment.

Anger May Disrupt Feelings of Attachment

A young woman may fear that her anger will taint her view of the therapist or provoke angry reactions that she could not tolerate—disapproval, a loss of affection or regard, and perhaps rejection. She may not believe that any attachment would survive undamaged, and consequently she may be inclined to deny anger to protect the relationship and her own feelings of connection. Suppressed resentment may take a greater toll on a relationship than would open expression of anger, however. Negative reactions can fuel passive–aggressive behaviors or emotional withdrawal, which may not rupture the relationship but may erode trust and affection over time.

Achievement May Mask
Underlying Self-Punitive Motives

Feminist writers have suggested that gender-related expectations can inhibit the expression of anger among women. Anger can be pathologized or stigmatized for females. If a young woman appears to be too aggressive or angry, she may be perceived as unfeminine. Chodorow (1978) proposes that a female's desire for caring and love can lead to a "denial of immediately felt aggressive and erotic drives" (p. 197).

Young women benefit from maintaining high standards and striving with passion. Competition can provide a healthy outlet for aggression. However, the drive to achieve, when taken to the extreme, can serve self-destructive ends. Such relentless effort can also serve self-protectively to defend against the emergence of inclinations and impulses that feel threatening or unacceptable. More specifically, the drive for athletic, academic, or professional perfection or domination can allow a young woman to deny feelings of vulnerability, dependent longings, and burgeoning sexual desire. Anna Freud (1975) described this type of potentially paralyzing struggle against "instinct and need satisfaction" as a "total war" that is "waged against the pursuit of pleasure" (p. 138). Caught in this struggle, a young woman may treat herself harshly. The self-imposed deprivation can become punitive. Self-loathing may be revealed when a young woman believes that she is never performing well enough or that her achievement masks underlying deficiencies.

Expressing Anger
through Self-Destructive Behavior

Teenage girls are at increased risk for depression and self-destructive behavior relative to boys. Such problems, of course, develop for different reasons in different girls and may be rooted in childhood experience. The conflicts and losses that adolescence presents for girls may trigger extreme measures to try to regain a sense of control. Through behaviors such as anorexia, bulimia, and self-mutilation, girls may compulsively regulate their eating and exercise or inflict pain on themselves. Such self-destructive behaviors and the tendency to dwell on perceived inadequacies may serve to suppress desires and distract from painful feelings. These types of problems have been described as "internalizing pathology" because anger and aggression are turned inward.

At a time when adolescent girls face new and potentially overwhelming emotional challenges, they are turning away from dependence. For this reason, a teenager may be reluctant to confide in her parents, thereby sacrificing a tried and true source of emotional support. She may struggle to deal more independently with difficult feelings. She may not, for example, even be aware of their anger. When an adolescent does express anger, she may not address what is really bothering her. She may act angry to cover sadness or she may cry when expressing anger, making herself appear vulnerable or weak rather than aggressive.

Self-destructive behavior may represent an indirect means of expressing anger, particularly to caregivers who are responsible for an adolescent's well-being (Perl, 1998). By hurting herself, the adolescent is inflicting something on her caregivers. A daughter may fear that parents might be hurt by, or might dismiss, her critical feelings. She may resort to self-destructive behavior to call attention to herself and her needs; it may feel like the only way she can communicate her distress and anger. In this way the self-inflicted injury may serve as tangible evidence of parental failure.

Inviting Direct Expression of Anger in Therapy

When therapists avoid conflict, they may reinforce a young woman's belief that her feelings can be destructive. Given the patient's fear of expressing anger, it is unlikely that conflict will be addressed unless the therapist notices and confronts signs of possible negative reactions. Therefore, by failing to pick up on unspoken signs of frustration or dissatisfaction, the therapist could easily collude with the patient's wish to deny her anger.

To address anger in the treatment relationship, therapists might need to consider that an exacerbation of symptoms or problems could represent a negative reaction to a therapeutic interaction. Similarly, a shift in the patient's approach to sessions (for example, increased absences or reduced disclosure) could also indirectly express frustration or anger. A therapist might, for example, notice that a binge episode followed a session in which the patient believed that the therapist had withheld needed support for her, slighted her concerns, or criticized her. In doing so, the therapist may confront the interpersonal meaning of the self-destructive behavior, thereby opening the door to constructive conflict.

To effectively encourage more direct expression of anger, however, therapists need to be genuinely receptive. This is no easy task, because it exposes them to criticism and possible loss of idealized status—or at least recognition of a shift in the patient's regard that would exist regardless. If a patient senses or expects that the therapist might be easily injured, she will be more inclined to hold back negative reactions, even if she is otherwise ready to deal with conflict. She thereby re-creates dysfunctional experience from interaction with a vulnerable or narcissistic parent who cannot tolerate critical feedback.

The therapist and patient each take a risk when they deal with anger in their relationship. By validating the patient's anger, the therapist acknowledges fallibility and may feel more vulnerable in relation to the patient. By expressing anger, the patient exposes to the therapist parts of herself that she might regard as unacceptable. But in taking this risk, each may become closer to the other, more genuine in their interaction, and more emotionally connected. The clinical relationship as well as the patient's sense of her inner experience are deepened and enriched. "Experiencing and even enjoying one's angry, demanding side often liberates a wide range of other affects, positive as well as negative" (McWilliams, 2004, p. 177).

Angry interaction with a therapist may provide new experience, gradually reshaping not just the therapeutic relationship but also the patient's attitude toward her feelings. "Expressing one's disappointment to a therapist who accepts this criticism and survives is an important part of the process of developing a sense of agency" (Safran & Muran, 2000, p. 101). This experience can then be carried into other relationships, allowing the young woman to express more genuine reactions and assert her needs and perspective.

Angry Attachment

Attachment need not be based on a positive therapeutic connection. The bond with a therapist may be just as important and therapeutic when it provides a safe place in which to be angry. By turning her anger toward the therapist, a young woman who struggles with depression or self-destructive behavior can protect herself from tormenting self-critical thoughts or damaging impulses. In this way she may use the therapeutic relationship to manage destructive feelings that would otherwise be turned inward.

Although potentially sustaining, an angry bond may not feel much like attachment. Faced with persistent criticism, anger, or a loss of expressed positive regard, therapists may lose confidence in the treatment or burn out, and consequently may withdraw or eventually overtly reject the patient to protect their own emotional well-being. To avoid reacting with retaliatory aggression or self-protective withdrawal, therapists must be realistic about what they can and cannot tolerate. When a patient needs to be angry, there may be no way for a therapist to work toward resolution of the inevitable conflicts that arise. Efforts to confront problems in the relationship or make insights may have little impact. Regardless of how hard they try, therapists may be unable to restore the sense of affection and positive connection that seems to have been lost (but may, in fact, still exist even though it is currently being denied).

However, there may be no need to resolve the anger. "Sometimes when powerful negative affects and enactments engulf both parties, there is nothing to do but endure it" (McWilliams, 2004, p. 177). Winnicott (1949) described the place of hate in a caregiving relationship—even with an infant. "The most remarkable thing about a mother is her ability to be hurt so much by her baby and to hate so much without paying the child out, and her ability to wait for rewards that may or may not come at a later date" (p. 74). Winnicott made a courageous contribution by acknowledging that an angry or provocative patient can have a powerful negative emotional impact on a therapist. He affirmed that it is okay for a therapist to be angry with a patient. There may be times in which therapists need to set limits to protect the patient, the therapeutic value of the treatment, or themselves. But often there is nothing that can or needs to be done about the patient's anger beyond the therapist's efforts to remain open to and engaged with the patient. Safran and Muran (2000) explain that "there are some situations in which the most important thing the therapist can do for the patient is to survive his or her anger or destructiveness" (p. 105). They proceed to suggest that:

The most important principle is for therapists to stay mindful and aware of the difficult feelings that are emerging in them as they experience themselves as the object of the patient's anger and to be willing to acknowledge their contributions to the interaction on an ongoing basis. The task in this context is not to avoid or to transcend angry or defensive feelings, but rather to demonstrate a consistent willingness to stick with the patient and to work toward understanding what is going on between them in the face of whatever feelings emerge for both of them. (pp. 105–106)

Using a Treatment Team
to Deal with Persistent Anger

Any therapist will have limits as to how much anger he or she can endure, especially when working solo with the patient. Consequently, the patient and the therapist may each need the support of a treatment team. In private practice, a team can be assembled informally when an individual therapist communicates and collaborates with a medicating psychiatrist, school guidance counselor, a nutritionist, a physician, a group therapist, or another health care provider.

A patient who relies exclusively on one therapist may feel too dependent to be able to risk expressing or even recognizing her anger. If she is unable to maintain positive feelings in the face of her anger, she will need to deny anger to protect their connection. Herein lays one of the many therapeutic functions of team treatment. With the opportunity for multiple simultaneous therapeutic attachments, a patient can more comfortably risk becoming angry with any one therapist (Perl, 1997b). Her anger might be contained within one therapeutic relationship, allowing her to continue to feel a positive connection with the others.

Therapists who are targeted for anger may need the support of other clinicians to listen to their feelings, offer emotional support, and perhaps most importantly, affirm their value even in the face of these negative reactions. Through the experience of other team members who are not so much personally touched by the patient's anger, a targeted therapist can retain a fuller picture of her more appealing qualities, including her vulnerability, which can help the therapist to maintain a more sympathetic and balanced perspective toward the patient.

However, therapists who are favored by the patient might be inclined to accept the patient's negative reactions at face value, creating a split within the team that exacerbates the isolation of the targeted therapist. When therapists are valued or even idealized by a patient, it is easier for them to see her favorable qualities and to take on her perspective. Consequently, they may find fault with the "problem therapist" rather than consider the therapeutic functions that this therapist is serving. Idealized therapists may fail to recognize that the patient is able to sustain positive connections with them partly because her anger is contained in one negatively charged therapeutic relationship.

Therapists Need to Hold On to the Value of Attachment When the Patient Cannot

Even when a patient insists that the therapy is failing her, she might be devastated if the therapist actually terminated their work. She needs the therapist to see that there is more to her and to her experience of the therapy than her anger would suggest. Yet, she may try to conceal her progress, making no mention of lessened depression or self-destructive behavior that might result from the opportunity to direct her anger toward the therapist.

When therapists continue to appreciate the patient's vulnerability and attachment, they demonstrate that empathy and care can coexist with and survive anger and even feelings of disconnection. Safran and Muran (2000) note:

> The therapist, by empathizing with the patient's experience of and reaction to the rupture, demonstrates that potentially divisive feelings (e.g., anger, disappointment) are acceptable and that experiencing nurturance and relatedness are not contingent on disowning part of oneself. He or she demonstrates that relatedness is possible in the very fact of separateness and that nurturance is possible even though it can never completely fill the void that is part of the human condition. (p. 102)

But if acting out continues or escalates as a young woman vents her anger toward the therapist, there is reason to question whether she is using the treatment to contain aggressive impulses or whether she is motivated by a wish to torment the therapist. She might be repeating destructive patterns within treatment, taking on the role of aggressor and inflicting on the therapist some version of what a parent has inflicted on her. The way in which a patient deals with her anger, relative to the specific sensitivities and vulnerabilities of a particular therapist, can reveal how she is using the treatment. She might be "pressing on" what she suspects might be her therapist's vulnerabilities, possibly deriving some gratification from the power. Alternatively, she might be exercising restraint to minimize the potential damaging impact of her anger. If she is acting from self-protective rather than aggressive motives, the patient might impose her own limits on her anger. She may not acknowledge her concern for the therapist, but it may be evident in her effort to respect the therapist's stated or implied limits and to use the therapeutic relationship to contain her anger rather than gratify aggressive impulses.

If a patient is angry but also attached to the therapist, she may be acutely sensitive to rejection. Despite her critical attitude, she may nonetheless worry about how the therapist feels about her. She may hunger for affection even as she provokes rejection. Therapists may begin to question their value or may just be too angry or worn down to continue their work, even if it might be beneficial for the patient. Following such an abandonment, a patient may be less able to establish the type of attachment with a new therapist that might allow her to express anger.

Now, returning to Sophia, I explore my own difficulty, even within the context of a treatment team, tolerating her persistent anger. I had been able to deal with Sophia's anger until she carried it into the partial hospital community, and it began to affect how I was perceived by colleagues and other patients. As support for my work with Sophia in the program began to erode, I reached a point where I felt that I would be unable to continue in my role as her individual therapist, despite the benefits that I believed our work was providing. This was a loss for me because we had been very much attached, and I understood that she was expressing only a part of her feelings for me. It was a loss for Sophia because she had relied on my ability to tolerate, and provide an outlet for, her anger.

From the outset of her treatment in the partial hospital program, I had been touched by Sophia's ability to empathize with, and understand, other patients. This ability probably accounted for the compelling influence on other patients of her negative reactions to me. Initially, Sophia related to me with warmth and sensitivity, as she did with other therapists. Her positive connection with other staff and patients continued, but with no apparent provocation, she gradually became increasingly angry with me. At first, her anger was sporadic, and we could still find opportunities to be playful and affectionate. Then these trusting moments became increasingly rare. The sessions became more consistently tense as Sophia slipped into a hostile stance toward me, and she began to complain that I was cold, uncaring, and insensitive.

I did not know what I might be doing wrong or what had changed in our relationship. I think we were both surprised by our immediate ability to connect with each other, and it was possible that she might have been trying to put the brakes on her growing attachment. But she also seemed really convinced that I did not understand her or know what she needed. At one point, I suggested that there could be a connection between her experience within therapy and her experience with her parents, who consistently failed to attune to her feelings. But my interpretation only confirmed for Sophia that I was unwilling to take responsibility for my emotional and therapeutic limitations. I tried repeatedly to explore with her why she was so angry with me, but she was unable to articulate any more specific rationale and seemed annoyed by my efforts to pin down a reason.

Sophia seemed unable to take in the genuine regard and affection I felt for her. She became convinced that I wanted to reject her. In fact, I was worried that her critical view of me could erode my affection for her, creating a self-fulfilling prophecy. Under the weight of her dissatisfaction, it became more difficult for me to sustain and communicate my regard for her. Our relationship became more strained. As I became more frustrated and angry, I probably became more careful with her, which likely reinforced her perception that I was cold.

Despite her dissatisfaction, Sophia never missed a session. And her self-destructive behavior was in better control. Although she continued to restrict food intake, she had not made a suicide attempt or hurt herself in any serious way in the months since she had entered the program. Yet, she began to compare me unfavorably to other team therapists, particularly to the newest psychologist, who was closer to her age. She did not, however, ask to change therapists, although she knew it would be possible to do so. I acknowledged her frustrations but told her that I did not buy the notion that her work with me was not valuable. I realized that she might continue to feel angry and disappointed even if I tried to respond to her complaints, but I emphasized that we could nonetheless work together productively. I did not point to the remission of her self-destructive behavior as evidence of the efficacy of our work because I feared that if I assumed any credit for helping her, I might provoke her to hurt herself to prove that I was ineffectual.

Over the next several months, Sophia continued to attend her sessions regularly and to refrain from self-destructive behavior. This was great progress, as previous therapy had never before broken into this pattern. Although she likely was directing toward me anger from other relationships, particularly with her parents, her ability to freely express negative feelings and show angry affect, while resisting self-destructive impulses, was a significant step beyond her past tendency to withdraw.

In the wake of this significant therapeutic change, she started to complain more vociferously about me to other patients. A clique of young women joined with Sophia in her anger. I was not surprised that Sophia had drawn other patients into our conflict—such collusion was to be expected when working in a group-based treatment program, and she had a lot of credibility within the community. Various staff members would become the target of anger at different times, so patient complaints were not new or unusual, but Sofia was particularly influential among her peers, and her anger was unusually intense and focused. Consequently, I remained in a more prominently and persistently negative role.

Sophia also began to complain about me to her therapist outside the partial program. This therapist, with whom I had collaborated well in the past, wanted to be responsive to Sophia's concerns and took the step of personally requesting that she be given a different therapist for her individual work within the program. My team members recognized that Sophia was doing well in her therapy and that she was beginning to control self-destructive impulses by verbally expressing her long-suppressed rage. Moreover, she had not asked us to change therapists. But when faced with dissatisfaction from this referring therapist, together with Sophia's persistent anger toward me, the team did not mobilize to oppose the request made by her "outside" therapist. As the therapy was already arduous, it was difficult for me to deal with any doubt from colleagues regarding my work with Sophia, and so I became less inclined to fight for her treatment.

At this point, I still hoped and expected that the partial therapy team would work collaboratively with her "outside" therapist to understand the split that Sophia was creating—specifically, why she might provoke other caregivers to react so negatively to her individual therapy with me when she had been doing so well clinically and was taking much better care of herself. I also wanted to use team members to reflect critically on my work with Sophia and to consider whether there might be ways that I could approach her differently. I was open to the idea of allowing Sophia to try working with a new therapist, although I was dubious that it would help and concerned that it might reverse gains that she had made.

Rather than feeling that my work was valued by my colleagues, I came to feel vulnerable with them in much the same way as I did when interacting with Sophia. The dynamic that took hold in my relationship with the patient was repeating within the team. For this reason, I became tempted to go along with the emerging consensus that Sophia should change therapists. I wanted some respite. Although I continued to worry about the possible negative impact of shifting her to another therapist, my resolve began to weaken. I believed that our relationship was therapeutically important, and I suspected that if she did not have the opportunity to contain her anger, frustration, and feelings of deprivation within our relationship, she would likely return to her self-destructive behavior. If we stopped meeting, Sophia would no longer be able to deny our attachment because she might miss me.

But my work with Sophia was costing me too much, particularly in my relationships with other patients and staff. Therefore, despite my reservations, we decided to shift Sophia to Dr. C, a young female psychologist on the team whom Sophia had experienced as warm and empathic. It seemed unlikely that she would form an attachment based on expression of anger with Dr. C. Once she was transferred, Sophia no longer showed her anger, and, for the first time, she claimed to be satisfied with her treatment. Nonetheless, about two months later Sophia decided to leave the program against our recommendation. Several months thereafter, we learned that she had committed suicide.

We could not know what led up to Sophia's death, especially as it occurred after she had left our program, but I suspect that she was destabilized by the loss of the opportunity to attach to a caregiver who could absorb her anger. When she was angry with me, she had been able to maintain other positive attachments. Not only did she lose me as a source of therapeutic support, she also likely became unable to engage as fully or consistently in her relationships outside of the program. Although I remained part of Sophia's treatment team, leading some of the communitywide groups, I could no longer offer regular, intimate, individual contact. Although Sophia seemed happier with her new therapist, the range of affect she expressed in her new individual treatment was more limited.

When treatment helps a patient redirect her anger away from herself, there will inevitably be some risk at any transition point. This is not to say that a therapist should never end a treatment under these circumstances, but if the patient depends on the therapist to deal with her anger, she will need an alternative relationship that can serve this function. Sophia might have been more self-conscious about becoming critical of a second therapist, particularly one whom she had previously idealized. After Sophia left the network of supportive relationships in the partial hospital program, she had therapeutic contact solely with her "outside" therapist. With the pressure of depending on only one person, it might have been too risky to express anger in this relationship, and she again became the target for her own aggression.

Despite the persistence and intensity of her critical reactions to me, Sophia was benefiting from the therapy—she had become less self-destructive. Her anger might have been difficult for me to tolerate, but it nonetheless seemed to be therapeutic. In this way, therapy can provide a safe haven for the expression of anger that enables a patient to better manage her feelings and impulses. But this is not always possible. In the next chapter, I consider anger that fuels malignant regression, possibly increasing (rather than reducing) risk to the patient. Within this context, a therapist's determination to tolerate escalating angry reactions and demands can inadvertently collude with destructive or self-defeating inclinations, creating an attachment that feeds regressive longings.

Chapter 6

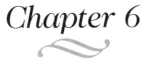

When Attachment to a Therapist Is Not Therapeutic
Recognizing Malignant Regression

*T*herapists inevitably invite some degree of attachment and dependence, which can open the door for the possibility of regression. One of the most difficult questions facing therapists in this regard is whether the regression represents a progressive step toward new interpersonal experience or whether it initiates a descent down a slippery slope of insatiable need. Teetering on the threshold between childhood and adulthood, adolescents may crave and benefit from a therapeutic haven in which they can indulge regressive gratifications—the opportunity to move freely backward might help them to feel sufficient control to more comfortably consolidate a stable autonomous identity. Moreover, therapeutic attention, understanding, and support may help to compensate for some of what a patient cannot or no longer wants to get from her parents.

But the regressive longings that are stimulated by therapeutic caregiving may become overwhelming for some patients. In the attempt to foster attachment, a therapist may break down defenses that a young woman has used to ward off suppressed emotional hunger, which she may act out in an escalating need for therapeutic care. She may create repeated crises, for example, which pull for greater therapist availability and involvement. With the resurgence of unfilled needs flooding the patient's therapeutic experience, treatment may become mired in repetition, and therapists might be rigidly perceived as a frustrating or disappointing parent. The patient may succumb to a sense of helpless dependence.

Therapists can provide opportunity for the patient to understand and express verbally what she is playing out, thereby creating potential for change. But the patient may not even be able to put her experience into words and may not be motivated by insight or understanding to give up regressive patterns that she finds gratifying. She may carry so much anger about perceived parental failures, for example, that she becomes entrenched in efforts to demonstrate a therapist's incompetence or indifference.

In the midst of such dysfunctional repetition, therapists may readily lose their clinical compass. It can be difficult for them to discern if and when the therapy might be tilting from therapeutic regression toward an experience of attachment that fuels self-destructive or aggressive thoughts and impulses. Moreover, it can also be difficult to predict whether, over time, the regressive repetition will begin to yield to new, more progressive experience or whether it will remain frozen in destructive reenactment.

Regression as Part of Adolescent Development

Regressive behavior may be part of a normative struggle among young women to assert independence from parents (Perl, 1997a). When a patient attaches to a therapist, this struggle may be re-created within treatment. An adolescent who is determined to defy the therapist may do so by willfully failing to mobilize her coping capacities, which can make her look regressed. Yet, in fact, she may be expressing independence by refusing to act in accord with what the therapist wants. The therapist may feel frustrated or disappointed, but this does not mean that the patient's behavior is necessarily self-defeating. A patient's willingness to forgo the therapist's approval can represent progress. It might be adaptive for an adolescent to manage regressed states, including episodes of stubborn, passive, demanding, fussy, clingy, petulant, or childishly defiant behavior by acting them out with a therapist, particularly if she uses this interaction to contain them. Moreover, these seemingly regressive behaviors may also function progressively to assert her will. In the process, the patient may disguise (from the therapist and perhaps from her herself) her growing emotional and social capacities, lowering expectations so as to reduce pressure to be more independent than she is ready to be. She may therefore benefit from continued gratification of dependent longings even as she develops increasing ability to care for herself.

It is also possible, however, that a young woman may be unintentionally sabotaging her ability to achieve her own goals. Her failed attempts to develop various aspects of her life—to find a romantic partner or to achieve professional success—may be a source of great distress. She may be troubled that she seems to be falling behind her peers. Despite her best efforts, she cannot seem to progress in a manner that is commensurate with her abilities, and she feels helpless to achieve a greater level of independence.

When therapists empathize with the patient's disappointments, without confronting her responsibility, they offer support but risk reinforcing a sense of helplessness that may confirm a patient's fear that she is a victim of circumstances beyond her control. Although she pulls for reassurance, the patient may need the therapist to confront her role in her failures—ways in which she may have systematically let opportunities slip by, taken poorly calculated risks, asserted herself inappropriately, or neglected to take steps necessary to move forward. By identifying self-defeating patterns, the therapist can begin to explore unconscious fears and conflicts that might cause a patient to sabotage opportunities for growth.

It may be difficult for therapists to be sure whether regressive behavior may be more adaptive than it appears and whether the patient might be more amenable to change than might be expected. Choices that seem to be self-defeating may protect against a more destructive alternative, or they may represent a

transition that helps a young woman prepare to take more difficult steps. The progressive function of apparently self-defeating
behavior may become evident only over the course of time.
When a young woman appears to be making poor choices (even
with the benefit of therapeutic reflection), she might, in fact, be
following a path that is different from what the therapist might
expect or recommend but that will carry her forward nonetheless.

I grappled with these questions for quite some time with
Serena, a very beautiful young woman whose passive approach to
dating seemed to undermine her goal of finding a man to marry.
When Serena entered treatment, she was stuck in a compliant role
in relation to her mother, which had held her back from pursuing,
and even identifying, her own independent interests. At thirty-
two years of age, Serena felt insecure with her professional and
relationship choices, unsatisfied in her job, and uncertain what
she might prefer to do. She began to date Jim several months into
treatment. The period of single life that preceded this dating relationship had been distressing for Serena because she was accustomed to having a boyfriend. To deal with her feelings, Serena
turned to her girlfriends. She also began to pursue more independent activities to fill in the extra time she now had. She was
surprised to realize that she could enjoy single life more than she
had thought possible, and during this period she was able to
explore her own interests for the first time.

Serena had come to therapy because she was so concerned
about her inability to find a man to marry. She had been unable to
accomplish the one thing that she knew she wanted. She had
cultivated long-term, committed relationships, but none with the
potential to develop toward marriage. Several of these young men
had not assumed enough adult responsibilities (for example, held
down a job) to be a viable partner. Serena, however, was most
concerned about her boyfriends' feelings about her. Sensing this,
her former boyfriends had taken advantage of her insecurity. Each
of the men she had dated seemed to become increasingly dissatisfied, critical, and controlling. Although she was annoyed by their
complaints about her, Serena would not confront problems in the
relationship or stand up for her own needs. Instead, she worked
hard to please the man and hold on to the relationship. By placat-
ing her boyfriend, she would become stuck in a relationship that

did not provide what she said that she wanted. She would remain dissatisfied but committed and worried about being rejected.

Serena seemed to carry into her dating life feelings of insecurity from her relationship with her mother, who did not recognize her talents and abilities or support the development of her interests or expression of her feelings. Serena would grow to resent her boyfriend, but she did not feel strong enough to challenge the power balance or seek a new relationship. She perceived her parents' marriage as a committed but loveless union, and she had no model of, or expectations for, finding someone who would fulfill her emotional needs.

I had reason to fear that this pattern would repeat in therapy. Serena seemed eager to please me, and she never questioned or challenged my input. I saw opportunity to exert therapeutic influence, but I was aware that I could easily fall into the familiar role of providing her with direction. She needed to find and assert her own perspective, rather than take on mine. Yet, if she were to try to operate more autonomously because *I* thought that doing so would be therapeutic, she would still be following my agenda.

It was also possible that Serena could not yet express her needs and negotiate conflict well enough to build an intimate relationship (with me or the men she dated) that could meet her needs. Her compliant stance could bring out domineering qualities in anyone, including me. When she got angry, she would become sullen and withdraw, expressing her resentment passively, with no expectation that her reactions could carry influence or make a constructive impact. She made it hard for a partner to respond to her needs, even if he wanted to do so.

However, it was also possible that she was choosing unsuitable partners or staying in stagnant relationships because she did not really want to marry, at least not at that point. Creating her own family was the only way in which Serena could imagine developing her life. And she pursued this path despite the fact that she believed that once a woman revealed her attachment to a man, she sacrificed her power in the relationship. She felt certain that she would repeat her mother's miserable marital experience.

By becoming involved with Jim, Serena seemed to be retreating from therapeutic gains. He seemed much like the men she had dated before, and he did not excite her even as much as some of her previous boyfriends. I confronted the conflict between what Serena said she wanted and what Jim seemed to offer. Serena had been working in therapy to recognize and deal with all that she had sacrificed to please her mother. Now she had chosen another man who was similarly controlling and possessive. Serena acknowledged that Jim did not support her newly developing interests, and she complained that he felt free to go out with his friends and family but would begrudge her the time that she spent with her girlfriends.

I felt frustrated when, out of loyalty to Jim, she turned down opportunities to date men who sounded to me like they could be better partners with more potential for marriage. But by opposing their relationship, I might undermine Serena's independent choice and fall into a familiar controlling stance. Whatever shortcomings Jim might have, he was still Serena's chosen partner. But I also feared that by supporting her relationship with Jim, I might be repeating her mother's failure to offer the guidance she needed to develop her potential.

I recognized that my frustration with Serena could be a sign of her progress. By continuing to date Jim in the face of my concerns, Serena was not caving in to my influence. Although I had not directly opposed their relationship, I had expressed some reservations. It might have appeared that Serena succumbed too readily to Jim's wish to exercise control, but she would find ways to defy him secretly (which was less progressive than confronting him directly, but better than conforming to all the restrictions he imposed). She was also less hurt by his criticism than I might have expected and sometimes voiced some of her dissatisfaction. Further, she complained to me quite a bit about Jim, which represented a departure from her tendency to become obsessively preoccupied with the man's perceptions of her. I wondered whether she actually wanted to stay in a relationship that she clearly indicated was not headed toward marriage as a way of resisting her mother's pressure for grandchildren.

By allowing the relationship to unfold in this way, I was able to see, over time, that dating Jim did not represent a step backward as much as a transitional experience. Serena did not take the initiative to break up with Jim, which would have been a huge step forward, but a year later, she did provoke him to break up with her. Soon thereafter she entered a relationship with a man who gave her more room to pursue her own life and who was more interested in her feelings and opinions, even when they were in conflict with his own. She feared losing her power to this new boyfriend, but she talked with him about it, and she confronted what she perceived as signs of his ambivalence toward her. Serena was working her way toward being able to feel that she could retain power in a relationship with a man, even one whom she liked, but she needed to take the intermediate step of defying my wishes and staying in the dysfunctional relationship with Jim to develop this readiness.

I would never have picked Jim as a partner for Serena, yet he served her development in ways that I did not recognize at the time and would not have been able to predict. By dating a man whom she did not and probably could not love, Serena was giving herself an opportunity to feel less vulnerable in a relationship and to practice more assertive and self-serving behavior when she felt she had less at stake. With the benefit of this experience, she might feel more empowered when involved with someone that she really loved. I have often been surprised that a young woman may further her progress even when it seems to me that she is making poor choices. At times, I might fear that she could be regressing when, in fact, she might be taking the step backward that she needed to prepare to move forward in a manner that I would have been unable to imagine.

Locked in Destructive Repetition

A patient may regress as she begins to introduce dysfunctional patterns from her childhood into therapy. Regression in the service of repetition may serve a progressive function, because the resulting reenactment can be used to identify, express, and understand feelings associated with childhood experience. As a young woman engages the therapist in these patterns, she may begin to recognize how she re-creates aspects of her past experience in her current life.

Davies and Frawley (1994, 1999) have written extensively on their experience with adult survivors of childhood sexual abuse, for whom reenactment of trauma might be central to the therapeutic interaction. Their description of the potential value and risks of repeating of dysfunctional family experience is particularly applicable to adolescents who bring immediacy and intensity to their experience of the therapeutic relationship, perhaps also with lessened inclination to reflect on their role in re-creating dysfunctional interactions. Specifically, a teenager might insist that the therapist is just like her parent, failing to recognize that she may be acting to provoke familiar responses. In this way, she may avoid responsibility for failing to access new opportunities within therapy.

Regression may reasonably be regarded as benign when it is part of the process of change or is moderated by sensitivity to the therapist's needs and limits. When a therapist is aware that change is taking place, it can be easier to tolerate regression, but it can be difficult if not impossible for a therapist to determine if the patient is actually making progress. Change can be slow in coming—it may remain hidden from the therapist, it may be subtle and nuanced, and it may unfold in unexpected ways. A patient's willingness to expose her progress in treatment may represent a gift to the therapist that can enable the therapist to stay emotionally engaged through difficult junctures.

When regressive behavior takes place in a context of mutuality, the patient may show regard for her impact on the therapist, perhaps by exercising some effort at restraint. For example, that which appears to be insatiable need might actually be moderated by the patient's sense of the therapist's limits. Or a patient might be inappropriately demanding but also inclined to show genuine awareness of the burden she imposes and appreciation for the therapist's efforts. This type of awareness and restraint must be differentiated from efforts to withhold their needs that are more aggressively motivated; a patient can minimize or deny her need in order to tie the therapist's hands.

But patients may also become mired in anger or feelings of deprivation, looking to the therapist to provide what was or has been lacking in their childhood family—often a setup for failure. A patient might resist the therapist's protective efforts and limits because she expects and demands unconditional love. Self-destructive threats or behavior may express angry reaction to whatever the therapist does not provide. Any therapeutic response will inevitably fall short of the unconditional love and protection she might have failed to receive in childhood. A patient may reenact with the therapist the experience of being disappointed with a parent, and she may be too angry to accept the help that a therapist can provide (Davies & Frawley, 1999). Therapists may become caught in reenactment that feeds regressive longings. When faced with the threat of destructive behavior, therapists may overextend themselves to try to meet the patient's needs. The attempt to remediate deficits in parental caregiving may interfere with the task of mourning all that the patient's family has failed to provide, "refortifying the child's expectation that complete compensation will be made" (Davies & Frawley, 1999, p. 291). The patient may then be inclined to use destructive behavior or threats to coerce therapists to reach beyond their typical limits. If a young woman is able to push her therapist out of an accustomed role or require involvement beyond the normal parameters of treatment, she may feel empowered to push for more and more. In this way, escalating patient demand and need can provoke more intense caregiving efforts, which can, in turn, feed regressive dependence.

Michael Balint (1968) recognized that regression could be "malignant" and, with this problem in mind, raised questions regarding appropriate therapeutic response. "Supposing the analyst is prepared to consider regression as a request, demand, or need, for a particular form of object relationship, the next question will be how far should he go or, in other words, what sort of object relationship he should consider offering to, or accepting from, his regressed patient" (p. 162). Balint proposed that therapists facing regression question whether the patient actually uses this therapeutic experience to " 'begin anew,' that is, develop new patterns of object relationship to replace those given up" that "will be less defensive and thus more flexible" (p. 166).

Mitchell (1993) describes the difference between malignant and benign regression. "Sometimes granting [the patient's] wishes can be disastrous—the patient simply escalates demands with greater intensity. Sometimes granting these wishes can be highly beneficial—the treatment seems more profoundly engaged than before, and things begin to move" (p. 178). Addressing the problem of malignant regression, Balint (1968) describes these increasingly exacting demands as amounting to " 'addiction-like' states" (p. 111). "A kind of vicious spiral developed; as soon as some of the patient's 'cravings' had been satisfied, new cravings or 'needs' appeared, demanding to be satisfied" (p. 141).

Davies and Frawley (1999) have observed the way in which they saw this malignant process evolve with their patients:

> The demands that were at first reasonable and uttered with quiet urgency become more strident and entitled. They slowly call for greater sacrifices on the part of the analyst and become increasingly difficult to keep up with. The relationship has, in essence, become an addiction for the patient, who must receive larger and larger infusions of compensation to be satisfied. As with any addiction, each dose stimulates an inevitable demand for more. (p. 291)

The therapist who is responding to ongoing distress or repeated crises may gradually lose perspective on whether he or she is actually meeting the patient's needs. It may not be clear, for example, when a reasonable level of demand becomes excessive or whether therapeutic interventions might heighten dependence. All reenactment reveals something about the patient's past family experience, and therefore may be of potential analytic value. But repetition in the absence of reflection will likely not be therapeutic, even if the pattern being reenacted has meaning. Therapists can never be sure when or if regression might evolve into new experience, and for this reason, it can be difficult to determine when it might be more therapeutic to limit destructive reenactment.

When therapists have consistently tried to accommodate the patient's needs, perhaps in the effort to protect their connection and minimize the risk of self-destructive behavior, the prospect of setting limits and losing her trust or possibly losing her to treatment altogether, may seem to be a greater risk. Because of this concern, therapists may feel pressure to stretch their tolerance, accepting a level of danger or acting out that they otherwise might try to limit. Therapists may absorb this stress and continue as a patient's sole source of therapeutic support in a high-risk situation, not because of any grandiose notion that they can save her when no one else could, but rather because of their regard for the value of the attachment. Even if the relationship seems to repeat destructive patterns, the connection may still represent the patient's best hope for change over time.

Therapists must weigh the risk of destructive reenactment

against the risk associated with the patient's reaction to therapeutic limits. Treatment may stimulate destructive impulses, and it may take time for the patient to develop alternate ways to deal with the underlying feelings. But it is also possible that the opportunity to inflict stress or demonstrate the therapist's ineffectuality could gratify the patient. These different experiences within treatment are not mutually exclusive, and the balance may shift over time toward or away from efforts to make therapeutic use of reenactment and contain destructive behavior. For this reason, the therapist will need to reexamine the risks and value of reenactment as the therapeutic relationship develops.

When I meet with prospective patients for consultation sessions, I typically am able to get a sense of what they might reenact as treatment unfolds and whether I feel able to meet their needs. Peggy was an exception. In our initial meetings, she presented as high functioning—a professionally successful thirty-three-year-old woman who struggled with depression. In an effort to assess the severity, I asked whether she had suicidal thoughts or behaviors and she assured me that she did not. When Peggy finally revealed her self-destructive impulses nearly a year into the treatment, I began to reconsider the meaning of red flags that I had previously noticed. I had been concerned about her tendency to lapse into silence during our sessions. I now recognized that at those times she was probably withholding disclosure of her suicidal thoughts and possibly underlying anger. Peggy might have been ashamed and she might have feared my reaction or protective steps that I might have wanted to take. As I became more aware of the severity of her depression, I became more concerned that the risk involved in the treatment was greater than I had initially recognized. But I nonetheless regarded her disclosure as progress.

However, as treatment came to focus increasingly on her destructive thinking, I wondered whether Peggy might be gratified by the experience of sharing these fantasies with me. Although Peggy's distrust most likely accounted for her delayed disclosure, her secrecy might also have been manipulative. I was deeply involved with her before I recognized the extent of her destructive potential. She might have known that I would have been hesitant to take on the case had I been aware of the level of risk at the outset. By this point, we had developed an attachment and a joint commitment to her therapy.

Because of her distrust, it had been difficult to establish a bond with Peggy. She was often reticent and sometimes completely silent in sessions. When I tried to engage with her at these times, she would give mostly curt responses to my questions. I sometimes struggled to generate conversation about anything. Initially, she disclosed only that when depressed, she felt that she was just going through the motions of life, doing what she needed to do while feeling numb and cut off. She explained that this cut-off feeling sometimes accounted for her silence.

There was a marked contrast between Peggy's inner world of dark thoughts and her presentation in her social and work life, where she gave no hint of her depression. This split reflected not only her strength and determination to keep functioning but also her ability to compartmentalize her feelings—which made it difficult for people, including me, to get to know her. Peggy was always productive in her work as a grant writer. She had dedicated friends, but they could not provide much support because they had no idea that Peggy struggled with depression.

I did not know why Peggy began to reveal the depth of her anger and depression when she did. Up to this point, I had been unaware of her propensity to engage in high-risk behavior. Peggy was single and had no one to whom she felt responsible. She now revealed that she would take off on her motorcycle, wearing no helmet, and speed recklessly along country roads. She enjoyed the exhilaration, but she was clearly flirting with death, which might have been a source of some of her excitement. In addition, Peggy would not hesitate to go out drinking at night by herself and would walk alone and drunk through dangerous parts of the city. As she described this behavior, she seemed unconcerned about the risk. Her interpersonal connections apparently did not prevent her from engaging in reckless action and harboring suicidal fantasies, and consequently I questioned whether our relationship could be sustaining. However, her willingness to reveal the severity of her depression and her inclination toward self-destructive behavior also suggested that she might be reaching out in a way that she had not in the past.

I appreciated her apparently growing trust, but I also recognized that she had intentionally misled me regarding the severity of her symptoms. In this way, she had compromised my trust in her and her belated disclosure did little to restore it. Now I was concerned about her potential for suicide—and I still was not confident that I would be fully informed. I did not know if she had a secret suicide plan (beyond what she had disclosed), how strong and emergent the risk might be, and what might trigger it. I did not believe that she would necessarily tell me if she began to feel less able to control her destructive impulses. I became concerned that I might inadvertently do something that could provoke self-destructive action. For these reasons, I was stressed by her disclosure—I began to wonder if she was gratified by the power to frighten me.

My interaction with Peggy became increasingly tense and centered on conflict, as was the case with Sophia in the last chapter. Both of them directed anger toward me. But in each case, the patient's anger served different functions. Sophia had used her anger to contain her self-destructive impulses and to create distance in our relationship that helped her to tolerate her dependence. She became angry with me after we had established a close relationship, and as she became more able to express angry feelings verbally, her self-destructive behavior began to recede. Peggy, on the other hand, seemed to use her self-destructive ideation to try to create a private, exclusive bond, which I feared might be stimulating her inclination to act recklessly. She was using angry, destructive secrets as the foundation for building closeness. In short, Peggy expressed intimacy by sharing suicidal thoughts. This for her was the base for attachment. It was only after sharing these destructive thoughts, for example, that she told me that I knew her better than anyone.

Soon after she acknowledged attachment in this way, she began to withdraw, expressing doubt that treatment could help her depression. Now she saw therapy as an indulgence and complained that she did not like feeling dependent. Yet, Peggy refused to develop alternative sources of support and consequently created the situation wherein she would be entirely dependent on me. She rejected my recommendation that she seek an evaluation for medication because she did not want to "depend" on drugs, but her resistance to such consultation compounded her dependence on me. I was concerned about dealing with this risk on my own. She refused to seek more help because she did not want anyone else to know that she was depressed.

Peggy might have been hurt and disappointed that I proposed

recommendations to manage her depression and reduce risk rather than simply allow her to share these suicidal feelings with me. I wanted to be close to her and I wanted to enter her emotional world, but I did not want to be her sole source of support. Furthermore, I did not want to tacitly support her denial of risk, which could have tragic consequences. But because I feared that I could so easily lose her trust, I tried especially hard to accommodate her needs and sensitivities. For example, I would sit with her in silence, and in this way I might have participated in creating a special, accommodating environment that was probably difficult for her to replicate in other relationships. However, she participated as well, drawing me in to an exclusive bond that gratified a possible wish to burden me with her suicidal fantasies.

As more of the sessions were taken up with exploration of her fantasies of suicide, the therapy seemed to become a forum for reenactment of destructive patterns. Often, I felt helpless in the face of her unrelenting depression, hopelessness, and despair. By revealing her suicidal thoughts while preventing me from securing additional support, Peggy might have been giving me a taste of her childhood experience of powerlessness.

I had been encouraging Peggy to talk about her destructive feelings and thoughts, including those associated with suicide, in the hope that it might help her understand their meaning and consequently diminish their power. Our conversation, however dark and disturbing, and my willingness to listen and to try to understand might build her sense of connection, which I hoped might also reduce her attachment to suicidal thoughts. As we explored this formerly hidden aspect of her inner world, her descriptions became more detailed and affectively charged, and I could not tell whether she was becoming more emotionally engaged with me or just more caught up in her suicidal fantasies. I became concerned that my willingness to share in these fantasies could be increasing their power. The exploration that I hoped would help Peggy identify the feelings underlying her depression and suicidal thoughts seemed instead to provide gratification— which I feared might provoke destructive action.

In an effort to acknowledge this risk and get more help for Peggy's depression, I decided to require her to seek a medication evaluation as a condition of her treatment with me. I thought that the medication might alleviate her depression, and I also felt that I needed a treatment partner. I could create a team with a psychiatrist, which might help to defuse our dark dyadic bond. Peggy was furious that I imposed conditions on her treatment. She agreed to the psychiatric evaluation and she took the prescribed medication, but she insisted that she would never trust me again. She believed that I had used her attachment to coerce her to do something that she did not want to do. Peggy was verbalizing the feeling I had experienced with her—I had similarly felt coerced to tolerate the risk she imposed because of her attachment to me.

Peggy complained that I had betrayed her. I noted that this was the first time I had seen her express anger directly, and I wanted to talk about her negative reactions. She explained that she does not like to be angry and she does not want to be involved with people who make her angry. She said that she had never before expressed anger in a close relationship, and no one in her family ever got angry. Her parents would dismiss any negative reaction she might express. I told her that she had probably suppressed a lot of anger since childhood and suggested that if she could express these feelings directly, she might be less prone to depression. At the same time, I was concerned that Peggy could feel so betrayed that she might act on her self-destructive impulses. Nonetheless, I held firm on my position with regard to the medication.

After several weeks of unabated anger, Peggy told me that she was quitting treatment. She had left therapy on two previous occasions, departures initiated, I believed, when she began to feel too dependent or too exposed in the therapy, but then it seemed that Peggy was trying to pace the work. Each time I had been quite confident that she would return, which she did weeks later after she had become more depressed. These breaks made it more difficult to do the consistent work required to deal with her depression, but they seemed to allow her to exercise needed control. The freedom to come and go might have helped her tolerate her growing attachment. Because she was so angry now, I was less certain that she would return, and I was also more concerned about her ability to manage her anger and depression without ongoing therapeutic support.

About five weeks later, Peggy called to make an appointment. I was unsettled by her angry departure and her failure to acknowledge our conflict as she made plans to resume. I wanted to give her room to pace the work, but I worried that I might be participating in a dysfunctional dynamic by allowing her to repeatedly interrupt the therapy by leaving in a fit of anger and then returning. When she would renew contact, she did not seem interested in dealing with our conflict nor would she acknowledge that she might have missed me; she would simply explain that her depression had become unmanageable. But I was committed to talking about the pattern, so that she could not act as though the conflict had not taken place. Her growing attachment seemed to be making our relationship more volatile, not more stable, as I would have hoped.

I told Peggy that I would expect that we would talk about her anger as she resumed her work. To some extent, she complied. She complained more vehemently about my mandate for psychiatric evaluation, but she also admitted that the medication was helping. For the first time, she acknowledged that she feared her unexpected episodes of depression and we worked to identify precursors and triggers. I was beginning to think that we might have found a way to deal with her depression more effectively.

About six months later, and without any precipitant I could identify, Peggy disclosed that she had a suicide plan that she intended to carry out in several months. She would not reveal the nature of the plan or the reason for the timing, but she explained that she wanted to understand why she had these thoughts so she could be "freer of them." I had been encouraging her to try to understand the meaning of her destructive fantasies, but in doing so, I increasingly felt like a participant. I feared that to continue therapy as usual and simply explore the meaning and function of Peggy's suicidal thinking, which had now apparently evolved into a plan, might deny the risk that she could take action even as we were working on this area.

For this reason, I recommended that in addition to her work with me, Peggy enter a partial hospital program. With more comprehensive and structured therapeutic support, she might be able to deal with her suicidal impulses with less risk of action. It would also afford opportunity to involve other therapists, thereby defusing the intensity of our exclusive bond. I acknowledged that she might need hospitalization if the risk became more acute or immediate.

My latest recommendation further heightened Peggy's anger toward me. She experienced my recommendation as a betrayal, like she did when I insisted that she be evaluated for medication.

Our relationship again ruptured. She became furious and she again angrily quit treatment.

I was also angry with Peggy. She rendered me ineffectual in my efforts to negotiate protective limits. It was true that these recommendations served my interests as well, by potentially lowering risk in the treatment and my own stress. But Peggy experienced any attempt I made to restrict her freedom to do exactly what she wanted in the treatment as a rejection. She showed no regard for her impact on me, and she interpreted any limits I set as evidence that I did not care about her. She was making it seem as though I wanted to end our relationship, when in fact I wanted to help her and, if possible, continue working with her (provided that she would collaborate with me).

I tried to reach Peggy by phone and left her messages, but I did not hear from her for almost two months. She did not make any effort to respond to my concern and did not contact me until she wanted to set up another appointment. At this point I was unwilling to pick up where we had left off. The risk had escalated beyond what I could tolerate. I had been too worried throughout her absence; although there was no immediate threat, she seemed to be getting closer to acting on her fantasies of suicide. I did not want to repeat this cycle, and I was becoming more convinced that, despite our attachment, we should not continue working together until she developed a network of therapeutic relationships. I tried to help her transition to a partial hospital treatment program where she would have access to multiple therapists who would be better equipped to work with high-risk patients such as Peggy. Again she refused this plan.

I had consistently failed in my efforts to incorporate other caregivers into the therapy. When Peggy finally agreed to seek medication, she insisted on returning to a psychiatrist she had seen several years before, rather than trying someone new, with whom I had an established working relationship. The psychiatrist she had chosen was accustomed to working solo with patients, and he proved to be reluctant to follow through with our initial plan to consult regularly. He offered only medication management. He did not engage with Peggy emotionally or talk about her current suicide risks. Consequently, the referral did little to reduce my sense of burdened isolation.

Peggy and I had bonded, in large part, around the threat of

her suicide. I was constantly faced with the risk of losing her, either because she would end treatment permanently or because she would kill herself. I felt coerced by the threat of losing her trust and possibly losing her. She felt coerced by conditions I imposed on the treatment. We were at an impasse. Peggy wanted to use our relationship to express and explore her suicidal fantasies. I could feel comfortable doing so only if there were some indication that our work was helping to contain these impulses. I wondered, especially in light of her growing dependence, whether Peggy relied on suicidal ideation to assert autonomy and defy my protective efforts.

I explained to Peggy that I did not want to repeat the cycle of increasing risk, anger, and withdrawal. Peggy would not consider including anyone else in her treatment—not a partial program and not a psychotherapy group. She would not reveal the severity of her depression and suicidal thinking to anyone but me. She explained that she would not permit me to bring other therapists into her treatment. She would not want to return to therapy with me if anything would be different in the new round of treatment. Instead, she preferred to work with her psychiatrist, to pursue all her treatment with him or psychotherapy with someone he would recommend. I was concerned that in this new therapy she would repeat the same problem and thwart the therapist's ability to deal with the risk that she exposed. Or, more likely, she would return to her reticent position, perhaps refusing to even introduce her suicidal thinking into the treatment.

I suspected that Peggy was using the therapy with me to re-create some aspect of her childhood experience, but she would not reveal enough for me to understand the historical meaning of our pattern of interaction. It was possible that the opportunity to share her darkest thoughts and feelings might have been sustaining, providing an experience of intimacy that she craved. However, I did not want to be lulled into a state of complacency and count on the fact that our bond could prevent her suicide.

There may have been change taking hold within Peggy that I did not fully appreciate. She had become more able to express anger as well as feelings of attachment. And it was possible that the therapeutic value of the regression would emerge more clearly if I had been willing to continue to accommodate her demands. However, after more than a year sitting with this regression, I had not seen signs of a "new beginning" and, in fact, our roles and her experience of me remained rigidly fixed despite my persistent efforts to create opportunity for different interaction.

A treatment bond that remains exclusive and central to a young woman's life is not necessarily regressive and may be emotionally stabilizing. When therapists feel helpless, as I did with Peggy, they might be caught in a reenactment that provides insight into traumatic aspects of a young woman's childhood experience—her own hopelessness, perhaps, that might gradually yield to different patterns of interaction.

Yet, therapists must also consider the possibility that risk is escalating and regressive behavior is persisting because they are not meeting the patient's needs. They may participate in destructive reenactments of denial or neglect by continuing to provide therapy with inadequate resources. By setting limits, therapists protect themselves and the patient from allowing for too much aggression within the treatment relationship. There is always risk that a young woman will choose to leave therapy rather than to comply with recommendations intended to contain destructive impulses. But therapy is preserved as an arena in which regressive influence is limited, and an attachment is not permitted to justify destructive acting out.

Chapter 7

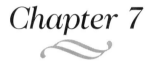

Beyond Idealization
Fostering Genuine Intimacy and Mutuality

Despite my wish to foster a therapeutic attachment, I kept up my guard with Kate, which made it difficult to fulfill what I sensed to be our potential to connect emotionally. I believed that her positive regard for me could be discarded if I offended or disappointed her. Kate was charming and engaging as well as a keen observer. With her poise, she seemed older than her twenty-eight years. She had natural interpersonal skill and sensitivity that allowed her to intuitively attune to the experience of the other, but she could use this ability to manipulate or control. In interactions with other patients in the partial hospital program, I had seen her cut people down while she remained cool and self-possessed. She was socially popular and always seemed to have a boyfriend, yet she did not seem to allow anyone to get too close. I wanted to understand this defensive position, but I was a bit cautious about confronting her. Although she had been consistently pleasant and polite in our interactions, I sensed the potential for aggressive verbal retaliation if I hurt her. Despite my role as therapist, I felt slightly intimidated and our intimacy was consequently limited.

A therapist cannot create closeness at will. Since I felt vulnerable with Kate, I tended to be careful not to reveal too much of myself. For her part, Kate did not seem inclined to reach out beyond our established roles as patient and therapist. She seemed to value my insight and respect my judgment, and she maintained a more exclusively clinical focus in our interaction. It seemed that her businesslike tone was designed to discourage more informal conversation. We seldom lapsed even momentarily into playful or casual chatting about something of interest that may have no apparent connection to her work. She showed no personal interest in me; she would not even inquire about my weekend or vacation. Kate appeared to restrict her emotional accessibility in other relationships as well, thereby also limiting her ability to express and deal with her feelings. I was not as inclined as I typically was with patients who seemed more receptive to personal connection to reach out emotionally. Consequently, Kate's defensive stance and my reaction repeated her central problem in relationships.

How can therapy help a patient break out of entrenched defensive patterns that limit genuine intimate connection? Given Kate's approach, it was difficult for me to engage emotionally with her. Ehrenberg (1992) makes reference to the "intimate edge" within the treatment relationship, suggesting that therapists consider emotional connection within the context of whatever constraints emerge in their interaction. Intimacy, from this perspective, comes not from an effort to push through defenses and amplify existing closeness, but rather from the joint effort to recognize and acknowledge whatever might be limiting the relationship.

By confronting such tensions or obstacles to deeper connection, including ways in which therapists and patients might feel distanced by each other's behavior or attitudes, they can work to create interaction that is intimate by virtue of being "authentic" (Ehrenberg, 1992, p. 39). Although it can be challenging to exchange direct observations and reflections, a patient does not necessarily have to let down her defensive stance or assume an uncomfortable level of vulnerability to begin to develop the relationship in this manner. Ehrenberg (1992) asserts that "the effort to study the qualities of mutual experience in a relationship, the interlocking of both participants, including a mutual focus on the failure to connect or on inauthenticity or collusion, can become the bridge to more intimate encounter" (p. 35).

A shared commitment between patient and therapist to explore and express their reactions to each other, to talk honestly and realistically about their relationship, is itself a form of intimacy. By noticing subtleties regarding the patient's behavior or attitudes that seem to create a barrier, therapists communicate their interest, understanding, and attunement to a patient and their wish to connect. "An authentic encounter *can be facilitated* by acknowledging the limits of what may be possible at any given moment, where ignoring these or pretending these do not exist precludes a more genuine and penetrating kind of engagement" (Ehrenberg, 1992, p. 39; italics in original). The invitation to the patient to exchange impressions about their interaction that otherwise might remain unformulated, unarticulated, or simply private can itself lead to new interpersonal experience.

Intimacy involves an effort to reveal different, and perhaps hidden, parts of one self to another person—to recognize and accept complexity and vulnerabilities within self and another. By relating at this deeper level, a patient might gain access to new or previously disowned emotional experience and capacities. Her sense of self might expand as she takes in reactions regarding her interpersonal impact. She may use the experience of another person to consider a different perspective on herself and what might be shared. "For some patients, the opportunity to discover that neither participant need be damaged or diminished by the experience or expression of positive feelings and closeness is as crucial as discovering that it is possible to survive negative ones" (Ehrenberg, 1992, pp. 40–41). Interpersonal intimacy therefore cannot be separated entirely from a process of getting to know and becoming more comfortable with oneself.

Idealization Can Both Express and Limit Closeness

Patients look to therapists for compassion, wisdom, understanding, insight, and guidance, and it is therefore natural to idealize them, and in doing so to express regard and affection. At some junctures, patients might particularly need to idealize the therapist so as to fortify their own sense of security in the treatment and their hope that they might be helped. When therapists are idealized, their feedback might carry more weight, and positive comments might feel more sustaining.

But at the same time, intimacy may be limited by a patient's need to admire her therapist. A patient might be more inclined to withhold parts of herself that she thinks might disappoint a therapist, whom she admires, because she is perhaps more eager to impress. (On the other hand, it is also possible that she would feel freer to expose vulnerabilities because she is confident that the therapist would accept whatever she might reveal.) Moreover, therapists who value the heightened regard may hold back more challenging or critical comments so as to avoid angering or disillusioning the patient. By being too careful with the patient's feelings, a therapist might suppress genuine interaction and avoid more difficult therapeutic work.

A patient who chooses to focus on the therapist's capacities and her own deficits might increase the asymmetry within their relationship. By elevating the therapist relative to herself, she places more distance between them. Rituals of clinical interaction introduce some formality, not necessarily because they reflect idealization but because they highlight the hierarchical aspects of the relationship. Some adult patients (whom I regard as peers) address me as "Doctor" even when invited to use my first name, thereby emphasizing the professional nature of our relationship and the associated boundaries and limits. This type of interaction may subtly constrain a potentially greater sense of intimacy and reciprocity.

Moreover, when therapists are idealized, they may feel that the patient does not see them as they really are. Rather than getting to know the therapist to the extent possible within the confines of a professional relationship, a patient may attend only to selected aspects of her experience of the therapist. She might avoid confronting areas of potential conflict so as to sidestep feelings of disillusionment, disappointment, frustration, anger, or uncertainty about her treatment. Yet, the treatment relationship might actually feel more solid if the patient were willing or able to acknowledge the therapist's fallibility or limitations, while also appreciating his or her capacities, talents, and strengths.

The sense of safety that a young child derives from an illusion of parental omnipotence may bear some relation to therapeutic idealization, except that the latter demands an effort to suspend critical judgment that would be appropriate within a treatment relationship. In adolescence and adulthood, such security may come at a greater cost to a young woman's sense of competence. This idealization fosters a perception that a patient has less to give and that a therapist has less need to receive, possibly making a patient feel that she might have little to offer her therapist beyond her assigned role.

In her psychotherapy sessions, April often asked me to weigh in on decisions she was making, particularly those related to her work, where she was having some difficulties. She would eagerly listen to any suggestions I might offer, but she might ultimately choose to dismiss them and follow her own counsel. On those occasions, I did not believe that she was rejecting my input in order to assert her own mandate for independent decision making. Rather, we might have just disagreed on some things. She might have experienced a sense of connection from asking me the questions, with no need to accept my response. I noticed, however, that she was more inclined to mention occasions when she did follow up on one of my suggestions than on the probably more numerous occasions when she did not.

As April's performance at work began to improve, it was less often a topic of conversation. It was evident to me that she was gaining confidence, expertise, as well as some savvy in dealing with the delicate interpersonal situations that arose with her colleagues and subordinates. At about this time, she told me that she was concerned about her dependence on me, which she believed to be excessive. She explained that she wanted to cut back the frequency of her sessions so that she would be forced to make decisions more independently.

I was surprised that April felt so dependent on me. Even when she was using sessions to explore her professional struggles, she seemed well able to challenge me and defend her own judgment. April would often make big decisions on her own and inform me about them only after the fact. Yet, she nonetheless felt that she could not make a decision without me. As we explored the difference in our perspectives, we realized that she associated attachment with dependence. She felt vulnerable because she looked forward to our meetings. She was not dependent on me in any concrete or practical way, but she might have derived a sense of security from our interaction or perhaps just my presence. She was eager to talk with me, not because she needed input or guidance, but because she just enjoyed our conversations. If April struggled internally with a wish to give herself over to my influence, she did not seem to act on it.

April also seemed unable to accept my regard for her abilities. In one session our conversation digressed to an issue that I had addressed in a paper I was writing at the time. From our brief exchange, I was impressed by her knowledge of the subject. When I complimented the breadth of her reading, she felt insulted. She felt that I was assuming that she would not be acquainted with a literature that she regarded as basic. I think she was projecting onto me her own tendency to view herself as less well read and probably less intelligent than myself. As she came to recognize that she was exaggerating the gap between us, she began to feel more confident in her abilities and we both began to feel closer to each other.

Finding New Parts of Oneself
in an Intimate Therapeutic Relationship

The "intimate edge" is not simply at the boundary between self and other, the point of developing interpersonal intimacy and awareness of interpersonal possibility in the relationship; it is also at the boundary of self-awareness. It is a point of expanding self-discovery, at which one can become more "intimate" with one's own experience through the evolving relationship with the other, and then more intimate with the other as one becomes more attuned to one's self.

—EHRENBERG (1992, pp. 34–35)

Through therapeutic interaction, a patient may access parts of herself that have been denied or disowned (Safran & Muran, 2000, p. 48). Such disconnection may be motivated defensively. A young woman may want to disown feelings that seem unacceptable, alien, or otherwise threatening to her sense of self. Such a defensive effort may cause her to lose touch with parts of herself that may be restored only through the course of interaction with someone who is more receptive to her experience than she might be. Her self-critical feelings may soften as she finds that another person can accept and even enjoy parts of herself that she has rejected. When others encounter parts of her personality that might actually be difficult or unappealing but sustain their love and regard, they might help her to hold onto different and perhaps even conflicting feelings about herself.

Returning to my work with Kate, I describe a moment of closeness that emerged unexpectedly in the midst of painful interaction, marking a shift in our relationship and in Kate's sense of herself. Up to this point, our interaction had maintained a largely positive tone, and Kate had seemed to respect, admire, and perhaps even idealize me. Her attitude toward me was likely influenced by her regard for the authority of my position as her therapist and as director of the program. I felt that our interaction was actually a bit stiff. We seldom ventured toward more personal connection in which we could temporarily suspend awareness of our roles.

This attention to power, control, and social position was characteristic of Kate. She chose boyfriends who tended to be successful, attractive, strong, even dominating, and she seemed eager to submit to the authority she ascribed to them. With no self-consciousness about implications for her view of women, she would assert that she wanted her boyfriend to make all the decisions because "he is the man." Her girlfriends also tended to be very attractive, formidable people (even though they might not be as professionally focused), but she took on a more dominant role with them. Kate admitted that she would not "waste time" with anyone, male or female, who seemed weak or vulnerable.

I was Kate's individual therapist within a partial hospital program that incorporated group psychotherapy. This combination of modalities was intended to encourage expression of a greater range of feelings and interaction, which could allow Kate to become closer to and more engaged with other people and also more aware of different parts of herself. This might be challenging for Kate, as she tended to be reluctant to expose or acknowledge any vulnerability. Her emotional struggle was evident only in her tendency to abuse food and alcohol and to act recklessly. In fact, all of these behaviors—eating, drinking, partying, and risk taking—could pass for spirited fun. However, she had suffered for years from severe bulimia (that is, binge eating followed by dangerously frequent vomiting) as well as binge drinking, habits that reflected her difficulty in dealing with feelings, desires, and impulses.

Several months into the treatment, I learned from her group therapist that patients were complaining about Kate privately, outside of the group meetings. The patients in Kate's group seemed to enjoy and appreciate her, but they also were becoming wary of the sometimes hostile tone in her critical comments and were reluctant to confront her directly. They feared that she could become aggressively angry with them if they challenged her. Based on my own experience with Kate, I also suspected that they were intimidated by the way in which she cultivated an impression of being in the know, even superior.

Kate's presentation also made it difficult to confront possible hostile undertones. While giving critical feedback, Kate might smile, for example. She might have been trying to soften a difficult message, or she might have been insensitive to the full critical implications of her comments or questions. It was also possible however, that she was trying to disguise her aggression. The conflict between her verbal content and her nonverbal presentation sent a mixed message that might have made it more difficult for members to challenge her.

In the most recent group meeting, Maria, a reserved young woman who was particularly sensitive to negative feedback, took the risk of disclosing her difficulties in school. Maria had not graduated from college and now, despite her insecurities about her intellectual ability, she had decided to pursue her degree. She admitted that she did not understand some of the lectures in her math class, but was reluctant to ask her professor for help because he seemed busy and inpatient. Her professor had said that the material was basic, and consequently Maria believed that her confusion was unwarranted. She feared that if she asked questions during class, he would think that she was not smart or hard working. So she persisted with unproductive efforts to study on her own, and she continued to fail assignments.

In past group sessions Kate had been supportive as Maria had described her struggles with her family. She had encouraged Maria to try to resist her inclination to indiscriminately take in her parents' criticism. Now, in an abrupt departure from her recent expression of empathy, Kate jumped on Maria. Rather than helping Maria respect and assert her own needs, Kate insisted that Maria was not going to "get anywhere in life" because she buys into her parents' negative view of her. There was probably some truth in Kate's comment, but it was too harsh, and Maria felt betrayed.

Kate's aggression might have been triggered by Maria's passivity. As a child, Kate had suffered from her mother's passivity, which left her unprotected from her father's drunken rage. She resented and pitied her mother. In her reaction to Maria—by humiliating her friend rather than supporting her—Kate could have been attacking her mother's passivity and identifying with her father's aggression.

In her next individual session Kate told me about her conflict with Maria. I was impressed that she raised the problem with me, but before I could say anything, she walked out, leaving me to wonder whether she would return that day or even for our next session. She may have been trying to avoid hearing what she feared might be a critical reaction from me, which could have felt like an attack. But Kate did come for our next meeting, which gave me the opportunity to tell her that I appreciated her willingness to share with me what had happened in group.

I also wanted to talk with Kate about her experience in group psychotherapy and in our last session. I suspected that she might be employing self-protective strategies she had used to fend off verbal abuse from her father. It was not clear whether Kate was aware of her interpersonal impact. I told her that I understood that she might have needed space from me or a break from our conversation, but the way that she had left the session felt like a rejection—she had put me in a vulnerable position, leaving me uncertain as to whether she would return. I asked about her motives. Was she trying to warn me to be careful about what I might say to her or else risk losing her? Was she trying to escape her own critical feelings?

Kate was at a critical juncture. She could reflect on the destructive impact of her aggression or she could return to her familiar, more detached position and become impervious to my feelings and those of Maria and other group members. She had demonstrated how, like her father, she could be reckless in relationships, but she had also shown capacity for critical self-reflection. To deal with her interpersonal conflicts within the program, she would need to let go of her intimidating, defensive stance. At times, her aggression had served her well, as she could be appropriately and even impressively assertive. But she could also run over feelings of others and exploit their vulnerabilities. She was struggling to develop more intimacy, but she did not seem to accommodate for or even tolerate insecurity or doubt in another person. She was always poised to defend against vulnerability through attack, and no one was exempt. Her ambivalence about this therapeutic work was clearly intense—she had taken the initiative to raise with me her problem in group but then walked out before we could talk about it.

I told Kate that I did not want to pressure her to talk about her problem in group before she felt ready, but at some point I wanted to help her deal with her conflict with Maria. She insisted that I thought she was like her father. I told her that I thought at times she could be aggressive like her father, but that she seemed to have more capacity to reflect on her impact than he did, which could make a big difference. I said that she seemed to be confronting, maybe for the first time, her inclination to exploit her power over another person, or perhaps she was becoming more uncomfortable with her aggression, which could represent important therapeutic progress. I believed that she had not intended to hurt Maria, but she needed to deal with her interpersonal impact.

It was probably difficult for Kate to hear me validate her great fear that she could be like her father. Recognition of any similarity between herself and her father made Kate feel as though they were the same. This black-and-white perspective, while seeming too harshly self-critical, might also have served as a defense; she knew, in fact, that she was better able to control her anger than her father was. However, she needed to grapple with the ways in which she *was* like her father, even though there were also ways that she was different, and she needed to take responsibility for her capacity to demonstrate similarly destructive attitudes and behaviors.

Kate took the initiative to return to group and deal with her conflict with Maria. Based on our conversation, I knew that she was genuinely concerned about Maria, regretful about hurting her, and worried that she had undermined support that she had offered her in the past. Immediately upon her return, however, group members began to voice the anger that they had suppressed the previous week. Kate was blindsided, particularly by Tina, her closest friend in the group. Tina told Kate that she did not want to be "abused" by Kate, as Kate had "abused" Maria. Emboldened by Tina's confrontation and the support of other group members, Maria demanded an apology from Kate. Kate did not apologize, but remarkably, she also did not lash out, try to defend herself, or take control of the situation. She stayed and listened to their feelings and reactions.

When I learned of the harsh reaction she encountered in group, particularly the demand for an apology, I was concerned that Kate might take a step back from the more progressive position that had compelled her to return and face group members. Specifically I feared that she might reject Maria, Tina, and me. Instead, Kate seemed to stay engaged, informing me that she would not comply with Maria's demand. Even if she felt genuinely regretful, as appeared to be the case, it might feel humiliating to be pressed into an apology. She then began to threaten to cut off her relationships with both Maria and Tina. I realized how much Tina meant to Kate. Still, I could not be sure that she would resist following through with her threat. Kate had felt so hurt by Tina that she might have been willing to endure any loss to inflict on Tina some of the pain that Tina had inflicted on her. She might sacrifice an attachment in order to maintain her sense of control. I thought Kate wanted to reject Tina because she valued her opinions so much that she felt stung by her critical response.

Kate conceded that she did care about Tina's view of her and she feared that she was actually abusive like her father. But just when she seemed to be on the verge of exploring her experience in group from these different perspectives, she suddenly shifted gears. She launched into an angry rant, tearing into Tina and Maria. She left no room for me to respond, and I felt at that point that she was oblivious to my presence. Then Kate abruptly paused and in a calmer tone observed that she never looks at anyone when she is angry. I had noticed that she had been avoiding eye contact, and I felt that she had tuned me out. Consequently, I was caught off guard when she stepped out of this self-absorbed position and turned her attention back to me. Kate seemed to suddenly become aware of how she appeared to me in our interaction.

Since Kate seemed more receptive and more emotionally accessible, at least for the moment, I took the opportunity to admit that, at times, I have experienced her as intimidating. In this way, I was confronting her emotional impact, but I was also exposing my own feelings of vulnerability in relation to her—a more personal disclosure than I might have offered in the past. As I was able to confront her intimidating stance, I began to feel more comfortable and closer to her.

In this interaction Kate was giving me power to make her feel worse about her aggression, perhaps because she felt guilty or because she trusted that I would not exploit her vulnerability. This was a new relational experience for Kate—she was creating intimacy by being vulnerable and open to my influence. I was beginning to feel more empathically connected to her. Because she was already struggling so painfully with her aggression at this point, I did not want to make her feel worse. Furthermore, as I saw the force of her regret, I wanted to back off so that I would not distract from her own internal struggle or push her to a point where she would struggle against me instead of herself.

I also felt sympathetic with Kate's position in the group. Members had banded together and ganged up on her, exercising power by drawing on their collective strength. Maria's demand for an apology, which was backed by the group, seemed coercive and deprived Kate of the chance to make an unsolicited apology. Moreover, if she apologized to Maria because she felt pressured to do so, she would be shifting from a dominating to a dominated position. Now she, rather than Maria, would be caught in a powerless, victimized position (as she had been in relation to her father). Kate acknowledged her distress and disclosed that she had been bingeing and purging all week to distract herself from these feelings.

Kate then paused again, looked at me, and seemingly out of the blue, complimented my new haircut. Although her comment seemed unrelated to her work in this session, it was strikingly attuned to my personal concerns. Several months earlier, about the time that Kate had entered the partial hospital program, I had had surgery on my scalp that had made my familiar hairstyle unworkable. As I struggled to adjust to the cosmetic effects of the surgery, I had felt self-conscious both about my appearance and my difficulty finding a new style. At that time, I happened to mention my wish to find a better hairdo to Kate, who, along with all the other patients, had been informed of my surgery, but otherwise I had kept my personal disclosure to a minimum with her.

Given the distance in our relationship, I was a bit surprised that I had revealed my personal concerns to her. I might have shared my frustration about my hair so that Kate would know that I was working on a new style and might not assume that I had bad taste. I had always admired Kate's fashionable appearance, and I cared what she thought. I also have to admit that I might have raised my problem in the hopes that she would offer some suggestions. She did, in fact, offer her styling input. I believe that Kate sensed my vulnerability on this issue. Her response was warm but matter-of-fact, helpful and not at all intrusive.

On that occasion, Kate had responded to my feelings sensitively and without threatening my privacy. And now, at this difficult juncture in her therapy session, Kate was again attending to my hair and indirectly to my feelings about my appearance. Her question about my hairstyle was certainly out of place in the session, and defensively it could have functioned to distract us from her difficult therapeutic work. In effect, she shifted from a topic that made her vulnerable to one in which I was vulnerable. She could have been maneuvering to regain the upper hand in our interaction.

Had I interpreted Kate's interest in me as avoidance or a distraction, I might have been denying the sense of genuine connection and support I felt. Kate touched on a vulnerable point, but not to empower herself. By reaching for a connection beyond our patient–therapist roles, she risked rejection. If I had shifted back immediately to the clinical issue at hand, as I had done when she had raised distractions at other points, I would have been rejecting an opportunity to expand our relationship. Kate was introducing something new about herself, a softer and more nurturing side.

So we shared a moment of delightful feminine connection. Although the conversation was limited to discussion of hairstyling, I felt a deep empathic tie. Kate's comments were thoughtful and gentle. I had not placed much weight on our previous interaction about my hair, which I regarded at the time more as an exchange of social pleasantries. But this second interaction felt like an effort to reach out. It caused me to look differently at the previous interaction. I told Kate that I appreciated the way in which she had responded to my surgery. I explained that I had not talked about my hair with many people, but I had felt inclined to talk about it with her. Kate said that she sensed that I might have been feeling self-conscious, and she reassured me that although she noticed the difference in my appearance, she would not have thought much about the change if she had not known the cause.

I told Kate that I had especially valued her suggestions because of my regard for her fashion sense. What she thought about my hair mattered to me. Kate said that she was aware that she could hurt and even intimidate people, but she had never felt that she could have a positive impact, especially not in relation to someone like me. She explained that although she does not really see me as an authority, she would not think that someone in my position would look to her for anything or experience vulnerability. I acknowledged that I sometimes feel vulnerable, as she could see, although I am selective about when and with whom I expose this side of myself. I told her that there might have been some therapeutic value for her had I tried to present a more balanced picture of myself sooner than I did, but I also needed to trust her more than I did initially. I recognized that I was opening myself with her now in ways that she could exploit. She had trusted me and now I was trusting her.

With the end of the session approaching, Kate returned to the question of how she would deal with her feelings over the weekend, given that her conflict with Tina was still unresolved. They had planned to go to a club together, but now she felt that she must cancel not because she wanted to hurt Tina but because she felt so uncomfortable with her. Kate said that she feared that she would numb herself by getting drunk or bingeing and purging, but her more relaxed tone suggested that her press toward action had lessened. She looked sad. I said that her ability to express different feelings and to make a connection between her anger and her impulse to drink and purge might help her to resist self-destructive action. She had already been finding a way to deal with feelings and relationships differently from how she had in the past, certainly differently from the way in which her father had. If she held onto the feeling of connection we had experienced in this session, it might help her to better manage her impulses. The following Monday, she stopped by my office to tell me that she had actually enjoyed her weekend. I felt happy that she had been able to manage her feelings differently and touched that she wanted to share this accomplishment with me.

Embracing Mutuality

Kate turned her attention to me in a moment when she had been caught up in her own distress. She was thinking of me not just as her therapist—as someone who was critiquing her in the moment—but rather as a separate person, with my own feelings and concerns. She wanted to connect with me. By attending to my problems, she was able to take a break from her work and find some relief. Yes, that might be a defense, but I think it was adaptive and progressive. Kate was using her connection with me to help herself deal with her feelings. She was learning to manage her emotional experience by reaching out and becoming involved with another person.

Had I turned to Kate for help or support about my hair because I suspected or hoped that it might be of therapeutic value, the same words might have been exchanged but the interaction would have been less genuine. I felt sufficiently comfortable to let go of my primary focus on her needs, for a moment, and attend to my own, which allowed for increased mutuality. I was taking a step away from my familiar professional role and allowing for a more reciprocal interchange that included my needs. Kate may have been meeting her own needs for distraction or relief by changing the subject to ask about my hair. She might have wanted to connect with my vulnerability as a means of seeking comfort or trying to deal with her own. Ultimately, my disclosure brought us closer. But my primary motivation centered on my needs, not hers. I also doubted that her primary motivation was defensive or self-serving. Rather, I think her genuine and perhaps growing interest in me helped her not only escape her distress, but also gain access to a nurturing capacity that could sustain her even in the midst of her own need for caregiving.

Chapter 8

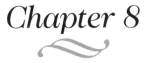

Repetition as a Path
to New Experience

*I*f attachments cause us to seek the familiar, how can we move beyond patterns that we have experienced in our family and roles that we have played? Such a question needs to be asked in relation to therapeutic experience as well as romantic, social, and professional relationships. I am not suggesting that all patterns are limiting or that we should break from attachments that may generally work well in adulthood. Rather, I am referring to attachments that may feel secure due to their familiarity but are preponderantly constraining, disappointing, frustrating, limiting, or have otherwise become largely maladaptive, at least in the context of relationships outside the family.

Dysfunctional patterns may continue to influence relationships in ways that might be difficult to notice. I may feel therapeutically successful when I begin to see new relationship choices or behaviors emerging in the lives of my patients. Yet, what initially appears to be a departure may actually cover subtler or more disguised repetition, or a repetition of a different version of the same experience. A young woman may free herself from a frustratingly familiar position in relationships (for example, a submissive or compliant stance) only to take on the complementary one (for example, a dominating or controlling stance). This shift can feel like a dramatic and significant change, when in fact it represents a different side of the same coin. She may not so much have moved beyond a particular dysfunctional pattern as switched roles, taking on an opposing position and thereby maintaining the same relationship paradigm. Yet, there might be some change taking place as well perhaps, because she is, after all, in a different position. Through this new position she may gain different experience and perspective on the other person and herself, which may lead away from the pattern altogether or at least add a new element to her relational repertoire. Particularly when dealing with longstanding attachments, change may not be only incremental, but also very much entangled with different versions of, and regressions to, the familiar. When a patient attends exclusively to what is different, she may be denying and thereby protecting maladaptive attachments. But if she focuses solely on what continues to repeat without appreciating what is new, she may deny her capacity for change. In this way she may take the "wind" out of therapeutic progress.

Kim, a very bright thirty-two-year-old Hispanic woman whose reflective capacities were well suited to therapy, struggled painfully with questions regarding her ability to create change. She wanted to use treatment to move beyond a pattern she had repeated since her first dating experience, in which she would lose her sense of volition and value as she attached to men who were older than she and in positions of power relative to her (e.g., as partner in a law firm where she was employed). It was possible that Kim was seeking the approval that she had never felt from her father. She even wondered whether she had become an attorney because her father valued his law career above all else. In pursuing the acceptance of older men, she set up a situation that would heighten her difficulty with asserting her needs. Despite her efforts to try to use therapeutic insights to make different choices in her dating relationships, she continued to feel unable to create a partnership with a man that allowed for a sense of mutuality and a balance of power and influence.

The twists and turns of this therapy led us down a path in which it would look as if Kim had broken through to a new relational experience, only to recognize a disguised repetition, but from the depth of that repetition would emerge glimmers of experience that really seemed substantially different. This example illustrates the ongoing uncertainty inherent in any effort to evaluate therapeutic progress. To recognize, sustain, and build on clinical gains, therapists must be able to identify change that may be concealed by apparent dysfunctional repetition, while also recognizing and confronting the persistence or resurgence of old patterns.

Seeking the Familiar in Adult Relationships

A young woman may be determined to avoid repeating her mother's experience with her father or her own experience with her parents as she sets out to establish adult social and romantic relationships. Yet, even conscious and deliberate effort to depart from familiar patterns can ultimately reveal itself as disguised repetition. Unconscious motivation may be in play here as a young woman re-creates in her social life aspects of her family attachments. Because so much of an adolescent's relational experience centers on her family, she may have had limited exposure to different ways of relating and may therefore maintain a restricted vision of possibilities, even as new opportunities come within her grasp.

For example, a daughter's childhood experience may have been shaped by her mother's anguish associated with her father's ongoing infidelity. As she reaches adulthood, she wants nothing more than a man who will be devoted and committed. But from her first adolescent dating experiences, boyfriends have cheated on her or dropped her to pursue a more attractive prospect. Because she has had so little exposure to committed relationships, she may not know what to look for when attempting to select a loyal partner, and she may be unprepared to identify "red flags" or signs that a partner might not be as committed as he claims to be. Her own experience may then confirm that she cannot expect to find a faithful husband. At a more unconscious level, a daughter's attraction may continue to be governed by her attachment to her father, even though he has hurt and disappointed her and her mother. If she were able to find a committed relationship, she might be appalled to discover within herself restlessness and an inclination to cheat on her partner.

Highlighting the tendency to re-create childhood experience in the adult "relational matrix," Stephen Mitchell (1988)
describes "our unconscious commitment to stasis, to embedded-
ness in and deep loyalty to the familiar" (p. 273). Mitchell emphasizes the continuing interpersonal influence of family attachments: "Operating with old illusions and stereotyped patterns
reduces anxiety and provides security not simply because the illusions and patterns are *familiar,* but because they are *familial* and
preserve a sense of loyalty and connection" (p. 291; italics in
original).

Repeating Dysfunctional Patterns
with a Therapist

In a similar fashion, a patient might be unconsciously drawn
to a therapist who feels familiar, and further she may act to provoke familiar responses, thereby shaping clinical interactions
to fit her expectations. Therapists' efforts to provide new opportunities may be overwhelmed by a patient's inclination to interpret therapeutic experience in accord with her past experience
(Hoffman, 1998, p. 125; Davies & Frawley, 1999). All that
might be different in the therapist's responses may fail to register
with the patient. Frustrated, therapists might eventually try to
forcefully convince the patient to recognize that they are not
really like her parents. But in doing so, they may inadvertently
repeat a dysfunctional dynamic—for example, dismissing the
patient's perspective. In this way, the patient's negative reactions
can create a therapeutic environment that becomes inhospitable
to new experience, possibly exhausting the therapist's efforts
to try to provide them. Consequently, their interactions may
devolve toward the familiar. Mitchell (1988) explains that the
relationship with the therapist "is necessarily structured along
old lines" (p. 289).

In fact, new experience may emerge not in the form of any
dramatic departure but rather as nuanced shifts in the fabric of
the therapeutic relationship. Therapists might highlight differences in their interaction with a patient, even while acknowledging a preponderance of repetition and accepting a patient's belief
that they offer nothing new. They may not agree with the patient,

but rather than seeking consensus or pushing for validation, they allow for the existence of both viewpoints. Therapists' ability and willingness to sit with the patient's need to deny the value of their therapeutic effort may contribute an additional dimension of new experience.

It is often left to the therapist to recognize the subtle and tentative emergence of new emotional experience. "The patient sees or experiences that the relationship can be affectively colored in one way only. The analyst sees more than one color, although the colors seem sometimes faint or fleeting—fugitive coloring that quickly moves back into one color, the color of historically held transference" (Cooper & Levit, 2005, p. 55).

Therapists create opportunity for change by providing an environment in which a young woman can be herself most fully and relate in ways that are familiar and comfortable, allowing her to reveal her feelings and vulnerabilities. This stance does not demand that therapists actually be like her parent, but rather that they invite emotional expression and familiar ways of relating. Using this attachment, the patient can explore past relationships with caregivers as they replay with the therapist, and in doing so, gain new perspective on old patterns.

The opportunity to challenge therapists, to complain about ways in which they are responding like a parent, or more generally to verbalize negative reactions can also represent new experience even in the face of the patient's conviction that she is simply getting more of the same old thing (Cooper & Levit, 2005, p. 57). A young woman may become aware of emotionally repressive influences from her family only as she begins to recognize the possibility of other ways of relating, which she might find, for example, in the freedom to voice complaints to a receptive therapist. Through this experience, she might become able to recognize the extent to which she has learned to suppress her negative reactions for fear that they would be dismissed or provoke a punitive response. She might have come to expect similar emotionally constricting reactions in social relationships. A therapist's invitation to express critical feedback could challenge her expectations regarding the way that people might respond to conflict. Such exposure to therapeutic attitudes might introduce her to relationship possibilities that she never could have previously imagined.

New Experience Can Be Embedded within Repetition

New experience emerges within the context of familiar patterns, and elements of the familiar will persist and mingle with experience that appears to be different. "What seems, at first glance, to be part of something old may also turn out to be part of something new, just as what seems, on the surface, to be part of something new may also turn out to be part of something old" (Hoffman, 1998, p. 186). Through their experience in the clinical interaction, therapists are in a position to notice nuances in a patient's relational style, recognizing what seems old and what might be at least subtly or partially new and different.

By reflecting on their reactions to the patient, therapists might be able to identify more specific relational patterns that are "rooted in the past and that the patient is pulling for in the analytic situation" (Hoffman, 1998, p. 186). By making these observations "palpable, vivid and accessible" (Hoffman, 1998, p. 186), therapists can help liberate a patient from re-creating self-fulfilling prophecies. The therapist's experience in the clinical interaction can shed light on the patient's approach to other relationships and her impact on other people.

For example, therapists might notice that they feel dismissed by a patient who never seems to believe that their comments or insights quite hit the mark or add much value. Further, they may identify the similarity between their insecure or frustrated reactions to the patient and the patient's reported reactions to parents who tended to disregard her input. In the clinical interaction, the patient might be displaying the more pervasive defensive need she has developed to "know everything," which makes her less receptive to input from others. This defensive stance could be self-defeating, as it might cause others to reactively dismiss her feedback or to reject her altogether, thereby repeating her childhood experience. In effect, the patient may be shaping the therapist's behavior to be like that of her parents. By sharing these impressions with the patient, therapists might draw attention to undesirable qualities she may have internalized from parents and identify a defensive stance that interferes with her ability to make interpersonal connections.

As a young woman becomes more able to recognize her role

in re-creating patterns, she might become more attuned to the ambiguity and complexity of her relational experience. Rather than seeing herself as a victim of her partner's controlling inclinations, for example, she might become able to recognize that she may be acting unconsciously to amplify the asymmetry in the relationship. She may recognize that what appears to be happening between them may be deceiving and that they are each shaping the behavior of the other. She might consequently become more able to resist the temptation to leap from an observation that something dysfunctional is being repeated to a conclusion that the relationship is the same as that which she experienced with her parent.

In therapy, a young woman can learn to recognize opportunities for new interaction. Hoffman (1998) describes the need to differentiate past experience from present, so that the patient can deal more realistically with apparent continuities between their relationship with parents and with therapists: "The content of the alleged repetition itself, when looked at closely, is probably not the equivalent of an interaction in the past, but bears only some analogous relationship to it" (p. 186).

Kim was convinced that her dating experience would inevitably repeat the most painful parts of her relationship with her father. Her failure to establish a romantic relationship had heightened her sense of dependence upon her mother, which made her feel all the more trapped, especially given her mother's own unresolved dependency needs. However, it was also possible that Kim's attachment to her mother inhibited her efforts to move on to a primary relationship with a man. Kim and her mother were bonded, in part, by their shared anger and the sense of rejection associated with her father's decision, when Kim was eleven years old, to leave the family to marry another woman.

Devastated by this betrayal, Kim had become largely unable to sympathize with her father's struggles, even in relation to her mother's neediness (which was also a big problem for her). As an eleven-year-old facing her father's decision to leave, she would understandably feel abandoned and also see her mother as being abandoned by her father. But this perspective remained fixed as she grew to be a young adult. She understood why her father might want to leave her mother, who was an oppressive influence in her life as well. But Kim continued to see her father only as abandoning her mother, when in fact, he was working to move on from a dysfunctional, depleting relationship—an effort that could have served as a model for Kim. It seemed reasonable that she might continue to harbor some anger and disappointment toward her father, but Kim did not give him any credit for his ability to move away from her mother. Caught up in her struggle with her mother, she had been unable to achieve even age-appropriate transitions toward prioritizing peer relationships. Kim might have benefited from identifying with her father's determination to pursue his own interests. She would certainly not have considered deserting her mother, as he had. But she had also failed to seek out other, more moderate and sensitive ways to break free from the protective role that she assumed in relation to her mother. Her anger with her father and her loyalty to her mother prevented her from being able to internalize her father's self-protective initiative, which she might have pursued in her own way.

Because she and her mother had been hurt by her father, her once healthy capacity to pursue self-interest might have become tainted. Kim might have come to place disproportion weight on the more potentially selfish aspects of this stance. She had not yet begun to separate out self-protective motives from insensitivity or indifference to one's interpersonal impact. As her father had moved forward with his new life, he remained oblivious to Kim's struggles and the burden imposed by her mother's depression, which had been dramatically exacerbated by the divorce. Kim's father was so absorbed in his own needs, particularly the wish to create a new harmonious family for himself, that he was actually critical of Kim's reluctance to embrace his new marriage.

Kim had sought therapy following an incident in which she agreed to have sex with an older man she was dating because she felt coerced by his power over her. Even before this experience, however, she had not trusted men. It was not clear, however, whether Kim was choosing men in positions of power who were determined to exploit their control, or whether she related to these men in ways that made it difficult for them to be sensitive to her needs or to develop potential for genuine reciprocity. It was easy to sympathize with Kim's vulnerability in these relationships, particularly due to the power differential. But it was important also to consider Kim's role in shaping the behavior of these men, specifically that she might be relegating herself to a disempowered position.

Kim had learned to suppress her needs long before her parents' divorce. Kim's mother had had difficulty managing the demands of a young child and, in response to what was likely normal childhood dependence, she began to refer to Kim as her "clingy" child. Kim's experience of men was likely also shaped by her unmet longings for her father's love and acceptance. Until she was in therapy, it had not occurred to Kim that her father's apparent lack of investment in her could reflect his own tendency to be self-absorbed rather than something deficient about her. Up to this point, she had believed that she was not sufficiently loveable to merit the attention that she craved.

Kim's father would ask about her life, but he would not become involved when she needed help or take the initiative to follow up on upcoming events. Consistently disappointed, Kim questioned whether she was expecting too much. She entertained the possibility that her father cared about her and just did not express his feeling for her in the way she would have liked, and she tried to find satisfaction within the limits of what her father did offer. It was also possible, however, that Kim wanted to believe that she was too needy so as to defend against the possibility that her father did not care as much about her as she would hope.

In therapy, we considered whether she might be choosing partners who, like her father, were absorbed in their own interests. With this understanding, she began to question her long-standing belief that she was too needy—perhaps she could find satisfaction with a man who was more emotionally nurturing. Kim resolved to seek potential partners who would be more responsive to her needs, and she began dating a younger man, Jack, a colleague who worked at her level within her firm. She chose Jack because he seemed to be emotionally accessible and even a bit vulnerable, shy, and self-effacing, particularly relative to the men she had dated previously.

Kim actively pursued Jack. She was taking initiative, which was a departure for her, and she was doing so with a man whom she would consider her peer. Despite their mutual attraction, Jack had been reluctant to take Kim out on "real dates" in which he took responsibility to plan an evening and paid for her. Kim wanted more, but she tolerated the pattern of casual, spontaneous meetings because she interpreted it as a sign of his insecurity, which reassured her that Jack represented a different choice. She was sexually attracted to him, but Kim allowed the relationship to begin on a more platonic basis—a departure from prior relationships that were initiated by sexual contact. Yet, despite some intermittent sex, her relationship with Jack did not seem to be developing. Jack did not even identify Kim as his girlfriend.

In therapy, Kim realized that she felt quite disappointed with Jack. Previously, she had blamed herself for her dating "failures," and she was convinced that she was "unlovable." Now she blamed Jack. He was too passive and hesitant to commit to anything in their relationship. Kim was making progress, evidenced by her efforts to establish a more symmetrical relationship with a more sensitive partner. But by shifting the blame for her frustration to Jack, she was not yet acknowledging her role in their interaction, specifically the possibility that she could be shaping Jack's behavior by acting in a manner that heightened his tendency to be passive. This would require that she shift from a view that their problems were all her fault or all Jack's fault to a view that they were partly her fault and partly his fault.

Moreover, to the extent that Jack did turn out to be like her father, or simply disappointing as a partner for whatever reason, this did not necessarily mean that Kim was not growing out of her old patterns. We may be determined to seek a new and different partner, and we may be ready to take on the emotional challenges this presents, but this does not mean we will be fortunate enough to find someone who will be capable of participating in the way that we hope. Luck plays a role in being able to actualize in a relationship potential for intimacy that one has developed (Hoffman, 1998). And we may need to become quite deeply involved before we see that the other person has some of the qualities we were hoping to avoid. In this way, repetition may be beyond our control. Kim was at a point in her relationship with Jack where she needed to explore what might be possible in terms of intimacy and what they might be able to develop together, given the difficulties each brings to the relationship.

I noted that Kim had been expecting Jack to demonstrate commitment, whereas she had been reluctant to expose her own needs, fears, and wishes—she was also holding back. For this reason, I encouraged her to express her feelings to Jack and to seek feedback regarding his experience in their relationship. I hoped that more genuine disclosure could build intimacy, or at least reveal more about their joint ability to move to a deeper emotional level. Rather than assuming similarity to her past experience, she could check out her concerns. Jack might be more interested in her and in her needs than she expected, and he might be affected by her inhibitions and frustration in ways that she might have not considered.

Kim admitted to Jack that she really liked him and that she wanted more—she wanted to go out on real dates and meet his friends and family. Her willingness to reveal vulnerability was new. In response, Jack said that he valued their relationship, but he did not promise any changes. Having risked rejection, Kim was relieved when Jack became romantic. She eagerly responded to his sexual advances, but hesitated when Jack would not use a condom. (He had used condoms on the few occasions when they had had sex in the past, but Jack did not like them because he felt that they affected his performance.) Kim was sympathetic with his discomfort, but she still asked him to wear one. She was taking an oral contraceptive but felt that her concern about sexually transmitted disease should carry more weight than his performance anxiety. Kim was thereby asserting her need in a way that she had not in prior relationships.

When Jack held fast, however, Kim acquiesced and proceeded to have sex without a condom. She might have been caving in to accommodate or to please Jack (possibly a return to old behavior) or perhaps she did not feel strongly enough to push their conflict any further and was eager to gratify her own sexual needs as well.

Kim and I reflected on the meaning of their interaction around sex. Jack had not been sufficiently responsive to Kim's concerns regarding contraception. He was putting his sexual needs ahead of her health concerns. If Kim had been more secure in relation to men, she might have taken a stronger stand, but her willingness to make the request was an accomplishment nonetheless. Kim questioned whether the personality qualities that originally attracted her to Jack because they seemed so different from those of her father and her previous romantic partners, particularly his "laid-back" presentation, covered a similar underlying self-absorption. Jack was imposing his will, albeit more passively. His more relaxed stance was not translating into flexibility as she had hoped. It would have boded better for their relationship if he had been willing to manage his struggles with his sexual performance and wear a condom because she wanted him to. An argument could be made, after all, that the use of a condom should not be negotiable, given the risks it posed, particularly to Kim.

However, Kim could have done more to attend to Jack's needs, as well. Kim was accommodating Jack but she was not addressing his sexual concerns or finding a way to talk more intimately. Jack might have been afraid of being impotent and of Kim's reaction to sexual failure. I suggested to Kim that she might have talked with Jack about his concerns (rather than simply agreeing to forgo the condom). We discussed ways in which she might reassure him, explaining, for example, that she would not judge his performance or be put off by any difficulties he might have. She might explore with him other ways in which she could promote arousal, and I shared some technical suggestions with her. I further suggested that she ask him to talk about his insecurities and fears as she reveals some of her own. In such a genuine encounter, they might begin to share vulnerability.

Although Kim had ultimately accommodated to Jack's wish to forgo the condom, she experienced their interaction as a negotiation and clearly felt that she was making a choice. This was different from her past experience in which she had felt coerced sexually, and beyond the sex, had felt a loss of her volition more generally within the relationship. And, rather than jumping into sex, as she had in the past, she had begun from a base of friendship. Their status as peers provided a different foundation for their relationship. Kim had become more able to look at men of her own age as potential romantic partners. Jack might be unresponsive to Kim's needs, but he could not exert the coercive pressure that someone in a position of power, such as a boss, could. Kim's willingness to question the relationship was also progressive. Moving beyond the assumption that she was too needy, she used therapy to question why she was attracted to men who don't meet her needs, why she makes concessions in relationships that feel violating (such as having sex without a condom), and why she might be reluctant to leave a man even when he is unresponsive to her needs.

Kim continued to repeat some familiar patterns in her relationship with Jack, but she was also breaking new ground. When familiar patterns began to reveal themselves, particularly when she began to entertain the notion that Jack might be self-absorbed like her father, she began to doubt the value of the treatment and her therapeutic progress. But even her complaints about the therapy represented a mixture of new and old. She had always tended to become readily deflated and hopeless like her mother and these feelings were re-emerging, but she didn't fall into despair as she did in the past. Moreover, her willingness to question the value of what I was providing was different—she did not need to protect me, as she saw me as being more resilient than her mother.

The persistence of some dysfunctional patterns did not diminish what she was accomplishing. To focus too heavily or critically on what Kim might be repeating (especially in light of all that was new) might also re-create her family experience. It would be like her mother labeling her as a "clingy" child because she cried and held on, more than her mother would have liked. For Kim, therefore, part of what was new was my interest in what was, or seemed to be, different and my understanding that any change would inevitably be mixed with the repetition of familiar patterns.

Using Therapy to Create New Experience of Attachment

Repeated experience is part of what builds attachment. There can be comfort and security in even dysfunctional patterns if they are familiar, and this comfort and security can create resistance to change. To explore new ways of relating, a young woman must risk giving up security for the "uncertain promise of relatively unfamiliar rewards" (Hoffman, 2006, p. 749).

A young woman may seize upon perceived similarities between her therapist and her parent (or between a romantic partner and her parent) as evidence that the current relationship is the same as that of the past. She may home in on what is being repeated to such an extent that she fails to recognize what is different. When interaction with a therapist reminds a patient of experience with her parent, for example, she may insist angrily that the therapist is just like her parent. By failing to recognize differences that may exist in the fabric of the therapeutic relationship or in the therapist's response to her concerns, she limits the opportunity to build on potential for new interaction.

Therapists may create new experience by helping the patient recognize what is new, especially when the difference might be subtle, partial, and mixed with much that seems familiar. It is important to appreciate *partially* new experience. The attempt to find a relationship that seems completely different may actually undermine a young woman's ability to recognize and build on partial differences and incremental changes. Efforts to reject outright any relationship in which a patient encounters familiar frustration may actually represent a lesser degree of therapeutic change than efforts to tolerate some of what is familiar and unwelcome. The ability to differentiate current experience that feels familiar from past experience allows a patient to "realize other potentials" (Hoffman, 1998, p. 125) in the relationship and in her own emotional and interpersonal capacities.

In the effort to avoid experience that triggers feelings or memories associated with past trauma or pain, a patient may inadvertently foreclose opportunity for new experience. For a young woman who has been sexually abused as a child, for example, the experience of being an object of arousal, even with a respectful partner, might leave her feeling exploited. (The same dynamic could hold true when the experience of exploitation is not sexual or physical but rather an emotional consequence of parental self-absorption or narcissism.) Under these circumstances, even an appropriate level of self-interest in a partner, manifest perhaps as he focuses temporarily on his own stimulation rather than hers, might feel like a repetition of exploitation.

The patient may not differentiate healthy narcissistic self-interest, in sexual or other interactions, from intrusion, a violation of her boundaries, and failure to recognize her as a separate person (Hoffman, 1998, p. 13). And further, she may be unable to embrace the part of her own desire, sexual and otherwise, that is self-centered. She might avoid adult sexual experience or suppress her own capacity for arousal by becoming emotionally detached in sexual interaction or by anesthetizing herself with alcohol. In this way she may be unable to achieve the deeper level of mutuality that could develop from a willingness to accept and embrace her own self-centered inclinations as well as those of her partner (Hoffman, 1998, p. 17).

Even as she struggles with associations to childhood experience, a young woman has an opportunity to differentiate her partner's sexual interest from past exploitation. The effort to talk about her reactions during sexual interactions might begin a process of differentiation, and the shared reflection might itself be a departure. Further, she might negotiate ways that she could take the initiative to stimulate him, so as to avoid the experience of feeling too passive, "done to," or like a sexual object. At the same time, however, she can recognize that even though he is excited and might be inclined to lose some of his focus on her in the moment, he can also care about her sensitivities and reactions. She may recognize that she now has room to express her discomfort and set limits if she chooses to do so, giving her a voice that she did not have as a child.

Hoffman (2006) asserts that the therapist will inevitably be drawn into re-creating familiar patterns, but that this repetition can serve a therapeutic function: "In attempting to traverse the distance from the old to the new, the patient may require that the analyst get caught up in old relational patterns—or get at least a taste of them—and struggle collaboratively with the patient to erode their power and to move beyond them" (p. 749). Hoffman's work suggests that any given therapeutic intervention will not define a relationship as being the same as one of the past, nor will it provide something so new and uncontaminated by aspects of the past as to be definitively different. New experience can occur simultaneously with the familiar, with difference emerging not necessarily from the absence of familiar patterns but rather from the ways in which the therapist and the patient deal with the repetition that will inevitably play out.

Attachments That Support Growth

When therapists are attuned to nascent or subtle change, they may make new experience seem more possible and thereby support a young woman's ability to recognize unexplored potential within herself and her relationships. She might be unable to find relationships that fulfill her needs as completely as she would like or that are as free from repetition of particular dynamics as she would hope. If she forms attachments to people who are rigidly attached to dysfunctional patterns, opportunity for meaningful negotiation and growth might be too limited. But if a young woman rejects anyone who shares unwanted parental characteristics, she may miss out on opportunities for relationships that might have brought happiness and end up too much alone or dependent on original family ties. She then might deny herself the possibility of interaction that would provide a base for shared exploration.

In a relationship with potential for repetition as well as new experience, each participant must take responsibility for trying to avoid playing into or provoking regressive patterns and for embracing and building on interactions that expand both of their roles and ways of relating with each other. For example, a young woman who struggles with anxiety might need to resist being drawn into a familiar protective role in response to her partner's intermittent agitated, obsessive preoccupation. If she allows herself to engage with his distress, she may become overwhelmed by experience that is too much like past experience with her parents. This does not necessarily mean that her partner is a bad choice or that he must find a way to suppress or control his anxiety (although some effort in this direction might be helpful). Instead she might need to learn to disengage or distance herself at these times, allowing him to deal with his anxiety more independently. In this way she might work on directing her protective efforts toward herself, which would also be progress. Her partner might need to work on accepting the limits that she sets—to tolerate or even support her need to step back from him at these times. Together they might thereby create a relationship that allows both of them to deal with their own experience separately while remaining committed to, and connected with, each other.

A young woman may need to work hard in relationships, including the therapeutic relationship, to resist re-creating the familiar and to find ways to deal differently with familiar patterns that take root. New experience that a therapist can offer will inevitably be mixed with disappointment and frustrating repetition. Therapists, however, can reflect with the patient on her disappointment; they can admit to their failings and limitations; and they can care about their impact on the patient and try to respond to her dissatisfaction. They can create opportunity to reflect on the interaction and give and receive feedback. Like attachments within the family, some of these more adaptive qualities of therapeutic attachment might be repeated in other relationships. A young woman might learn to seek a partner who can reflect, explore feelings, and connect empathically, like her therapist, and she can work to provide some of the empathic support in social relationships that she has received from her therapist.

However, the therapist is in the role of an emotional caregiver and can therefore focus on the needs of the patient in a way that cannot be expected in reciprocal relationships with peers (Hoffman, 1998, p. 258). A young woman might model aspects of the therapist's behavior as she takes on adult caregiving roles and as she attends to the emotional needs of her social partners. But if she looks to peers for the emotional attention she received from her therapist, she will likely be disappointed. Social relations offer the opportunity for mutuality, which plays a much more minor role in the therapeutic relationship. To enjoy the gratifications of reciprocity, a young woman must let go of the wish for the consistent attention and empathic connection that she may get from her therapist.

Based on her experience with her therapist, however, she may place more importance on the ability of the other person to both challenge and accept her. She may also take in some of these qualities from her therapist, much as she internalized parental behaviors and attitudes. With such shared commitment to self-reflection in her social and romantic relationships, the elements of dysfunction that emerge can be recognized and addressed in a manner that is gentler, more responsive, and even humorous.

Chapter 9

~

*Allowing for Attachment
after Therapy Ends*

*B*elle had never allowed herself to rely on relationships for support, and she tended to suppress her emotional needs. Exceptionally thin, strong, and athletic at 28 years of age, Belle was a former state gymnastics champion, accustomed to challenge and physical adversity. Her anorexia and tendency toward self-deprivation seemed adaptive within this context, as did her inclination to push herself beyond healthy limits and ignore physical pain. These emotional attributes that had brought her competitive success also reflected a serious level of disregard for her needs, both physical and emotional.

In gymnastics, Belle seemed to have found an outlet for her anger and self-punitive inclinations but more than that, her suppressed anger became fuel for achievement. Despite the opportunity to channel her aggression outward through competition, she also turned these impulses inward—since adolescence she had cut her arms and fasted and vomited for "weight control." I also believed that she was unconsciously driven to push herself in sports to the point of injury. For Belle, the line between self-destruction and achievement was thin, and she was even more attached to these patterns because they had served her so well. She had enjoyed both her success and the opportunity to recklessly push herself.

After Belle's eating disorder had escalated to a point where her health was endangered, her individual therapist referred Belle to a partial hospital program. They planned to continue their therapeutic work, using the structure of a full-day intensive treatment program to help Belle contain her destructive impulses. Belle had worked hard on these issues in the partial program and, because she had been able to participate in her treatment for several months without hurting herself, she felt that she was ready to think about leaving. Although I recognized Belle's progress, I questioned this decision. It had appeared that she was beginning to take better care of herself, but she had not yet begun to develop supportive relationships—outside of group time she kept to herself. Without regular access to a therapeutic community where she would deal with feelings and maintain social connections, Belle might regress to a state of isolated self-deprivation. She had internalized the capacity for self-reflection and emotional awareness, but she had not yet shown a capacity to cultivate mutually supportive relationships.

Because Belle was secretive, I continued to worry that she could be concealing destructive behavior. The progress that she had made expressing her feelings, especially anger, and asserting her needs helped to relieve my concerns, but only to a point. When she wore long sleeves on a hot day, for example, I wondered whether she might be covering self-inflicted cuts. It was also possible that Belle, who was acutely aware of my doubts about her readiness to leave the program, could be acting in a manner designed to provoke my concern because she was angry that I continued to question her capacity for self-care. Although I remained suspicious, I was also aware that Belle had been taking increasing initiative to talk about difficult feelings and issues in therapy.

As I grappled with the question of termination, I tried to balance my concern about the potential impact of a loss of structured therapeutic support against the value of acknowledging Belle's progress and respecting her judgment regarding her ability to manage on her own. Above all, I did not want to undermine her sense of autonomy in our relationship. From a practical perspective, Belle was determined to do what she wanted to do, and she would likely find a way to defeat any pressure I imposed that was not in line with her goals. Moreover, she admitted that she was not ready to end treatment altogether, and was clear about her commitment to continuing her individual psychotherapy outside of the program.

It is not uncommon for therapists to find themselves in the position I was in with Belle—wanting to go further with treatment than a patient might be inclined to do. Therapists might need to consider what a patient has or has not accomplished in therapy and how she is likely to manage without it, but a patient's feeling of readiness might be a more important consideration. A young woman's intent to leave her therapist also represents an expression of autonomy. Therapists might reasonably oppose this initiative if they believe that it would likely endanger the patient or cause her to lose gains that she has not yet solidified. But by trying to hold on when the patient wants to leave, the therapist risks repeating dysfunctional elements of the daughter's struggle to separate from parents. If she stays in therapy and even if she's feeling completely free to express her reactions to the decision, the cost to her sense of independence might compromise the value of potential therapeutic gains.

Because therapy is at the core an attachment, it might never reach a natural end point. An adolescent's need to move away for college, an internship, or a job may force a conclusion to the work, and therapy can focus on helping her to separate at whatever point she needs to leave. But this does not necessarily mean that the therapeutic work is done or even that she will feel entirely ready. The ending of therapy is like launching from the bond with parents. A young woman will always need emotional caretaking and attachment, even through adulthood. And the need for connection to a caregiver may persist even as an adolescent becomes increasingly able to care for herself. A young woman may want to move on from therapy, and she may feel prepared to find other ways to meet her emotional needs, perhaps not in relationships designated for caregiving but in supportive peer connections. Daughters turn from parents to peers not because they no longer have need for their emotional care, but because they are ready to give to others and to get their needs met in the context of more reciprocal relationships. A therapeutic bond does not represent the same kind of attachment, of course, nor is there the expectation that the balance of nurturing will shift toward the caregiver over the course of a lifetime, as there might be in relation to an aging parent.

Nonetheless, a sense of therapeutic attachment may endure long after sessions have ended. A young recently married woman who had just begun to think of stopping therapy as part of her plan to move to a distant suburb and have a baby told me that she could imagine coming back to see me in five years if something was troubling her or just to "check in." I was delighted not only because of my attachment to her, but because she could imagine being sustained by her attachment to me even after stopping therapy. Increasingly, our relationship was becoming part of a larger network of meaningful connections. She had been deepening her friendships, she was confiding more in her husband, and she had joined with colleagues to form a small professional company. In each of these relational contexts, she would find a different balance of giving and receiving. Her sense of herself had been enhanced from the growing array of opportunities to actualize her own capacity to nurture. I further recognized that her ability to think about returning years later might have suggested her increasing readiness to leave, as she was able to anticipate possible needs, think in terms of seeking support, and internalize a sense of attachment to me that could survive without direct contact.

Using a Therapist as a Base for "Refueling"

As is the case with parents and adolescent daughters, healthy separation from therapists is supported by the opportunity for continued connection. By inviting contact after "termination" and maintaining continued interest in the patient, therapists can provide a secure base for "refueling" (Mahler, Pine and Bergman, 1975, p. 69). Whether or not a patient chooses to pursue further therapeutic contact, she can feel comforted by the therapist's continuing availability and by her sense that the therapist will remember and remain invested in her. Eichler (2006) describes the way that college students can make use of therapists in university counseling centers for refueling by seeking contact as needed. He emphasizes that a therapeutic plan demanding long-term commitment to regular sessions may not meet this developmental need as well as a more flexible approach that allows students to come as they see fit. Eichler explains the developmental rationale for this approach:

> Intermittent treatment is often more than just an accommodation to students' ambivalence. At times, it is the optimal complement to their efforts at individuation. Just as toddlers taking their first steps literally and figuratively check back to reassure themselves of their caregiver's continued presence (Mahler, Pine and Bergman, 1975), college students best venture into the wider world of new experiences when confident of a secure home base to fall back upon in a crisis. Students who drop in and out of counseling sometimes are not so much resistant or ambivalent as they are adaptive in using their attachment to the therapist to support their development. Long gaps in treatment do not necessarily imply gaps in the therapeutic relationship, which may be very much alive for students during their absences from treatment. Students may draw sustenance from their therapists' constancy and ongoing availability, the knowledge that they are there to be found again when needed. (pp. 29–30)

Therefore, the traditional commitment to regular meetings up to a point of termination may be particularly ill-suited to the needs of an adolescent and young adult population. In keeping with her efforts to exercise autonomy, an adolescent might need to regulate whether and how she uses therapy in response to her changing needs. She may remain in therapy until she feels less distressed, return at a future point to check in, meet a few times to deal with a particular problem or issue, or resume even more intensive and extended work. It is possible that she may use therapy sporadically, as needed, for years.

The opportunity to sustain attachment may itself serve important developmental needs during an ongoing therapy and also after a treatment is terminated. Posttreatment contact can be as therapeutic as regular therapy sessions. To the extent that a young woman feels that the therapist is invested in her independent growth, she may want to find ways to continue to share elements of her life "after therapy." Although therapists need to maintain their role as therapists, as treatment continues or in posttreatment meetings the interaction may appropriately become a bit less hierarchical with less expectation of clinical guidance.

After treatment ends, patients may be seeking an opportunity to experience an increased sense of mutuality with the therapist. A therapist's efforts to draw the patient back into deeper clinical work might feel like a threat to the separation and autonomy she has achieved. Here, too, there are parallels to the process of separating from parents. A young woman may no longer need advice or "parenting" from her parents just as she may no longer need analytic input or "therapy" from her therapist. But this will not diminish her need for the caregiving relationships, particularly for the caregiver's continued availability and interest in her life.

When Is a Patient Ready to Leave Her Therapist?

Rather than thinking of termination as a fixed end of treatment, it can be more useful to think of it in terms of fostering the patient's increasing autonomy from the therapist. From this perspective, termination raises the question of what a patient might need to do or accomplish to be able to function comfortably without the therapist (even if the therapist remains available to her). Planning for termination may, for some young women, be an important part of the process of establishing independence. A patient may feel that she needs to leave therapy to fully experience and demonstrate her autonomy.

But if therapists regard termination as a point of completion, they may be failing to appreciate the full scope of the therapeutic relationship. As was discussed in Chapter 1, ongoing attachment to a caregiver can be critically important for adolescent development. If therapists regard subsequent therapeutic need as a failure, they risk discouraging follow-up contact. Emphasis on termination as a goal may thereby undermine a patient's ability to make use of the therapist for emotional refueling. As is the case in relation to her parents, an emerging adult may no longer need any concrete guidance or help from a therapist, but this does not necessarily diminish the importance of her attachment.

Therapists cannot know when a patient is "done" with treatment and what continued use she might make of their relationship. Any ending will necessarily be, to some extent, arbitrary.

Mitchell asserts that "there is always more to learn; there are always ways in which the analyst and the analytic process could continue to enrich experience" (1993, p. 229). Therapy can help prepare a young woman to deal with new problems or challenges as well as new versions of old problems. Although supportive peer relationships can reduce dependence on a therapist, they do not eliminate potential need for what a therapist can provide.

But, like the experience of leaving parents to live independently, launching from therapy can provide an opportunity for growth that can be achieved only by separating. While in treatment, a patient may begin to make her own insights, engage in her own process of reflection, and apply what she has learned in sessions outside of therapy. But this is not the same as the experience of dealing with life apart from a therapeutic process. "One of the startling realizations upon leaving analysis is the sense that one is now fully responsible for one's life. The suspension that analysis provides, useful, necessary, enriching, is now over" (Mitchell, 1993, p. 229). Ending treatment can allow for a fuller experience of autonomy—but this does not imply that a young woman has been dependent on her therapist. Rather, her experience might have been influenced by the opportunity to talk about and "work on" her life as it is happening. Because therapy is about change, it puts in the foreground the sense of potential. Effort to pursue growth can and should persist after therapy ends, but it will no longer be supported by the formal structure and process that treatment provides.

So how does a patient know when to leave? Although it can be helpful for certain social and emotional developments to be in place, there really are no objective indicators of readiness. A young woman may or may not be prepared to end therapy when her "symptoms" have been relieved or when she has made desired progress on her treatment goals. She may no longer rely on the therapist for guidance or insight, and she may have other sources of emotional support, but it still may not be in her best interest to let go of planned contact with the therapist. If she believes that she should leave treatment because she has reached a particular milestone, rather than because she feels ready, she might consciously or unconsciously undermine her progress and even regress in the service of protecting her therapy.

A patient may be doing as well as she is because of ongoing

therapeutic contact and without the therapist, these gains could be lost. A therapist cannot know how much the patient's progress is sustained by their meetings. Although a patient could want to leave treatment for defensive reasons, her interest in, motivation for, and comfort with the idea of ending, rather than an independent evaluation on the part of the therapist, should carry the most weight. Moreover, the freedom to exercise control—initiating and pacing separation—is crucial when an adolescent is launching from parents and therapists.

Therapy may provide opportunity to work through difficulties encountered in the effort to launch from family, particularly ambivalent parental reactions to their daughter's growing autonomy. By following the patient's lead and picking up on her interest in beginning to think about leaving, therapists might be able provide a different experience with separation, in which an adolescent's needs will carry more weight relative to the needs of a caregiver, who might be reluctant to let go.

A Patient May Feel More Prepared to Leave Treatment When She Has Internalized Aspects of the Therapist and the Therapy

Particularly when she is attached to her therapist, a young woman may consider or imagine the therapist's perspective on life events that transpire between sessions. She might also engage in the therapeutic process independently by reflecting on her feelings, reactions, and relationships, much in the way that she does with her therapist. She might, for example, begin to consider her role in problems that come up during the week and consequently become more receptive to critical feedback. In this way, she can carry therapeutic influence into family, social, and work relationships.

Over time, a young woman may become more comfortable with therapeutic behaviors and attitudes. She might be more able to recognize and break from dysfunctional patterns and incorporate new ways of relating. For example, she might try to empathize with a friend in a manner similar to the way that her therapist would respond to her feelings. In this effort, she might utilize interpersonal skills that she has learned in her treatment. To this end, she must resist the inclination to fall back into more familiar and comfortable patterns of relating that might cause her, for example, to take on an opinionated or directive position with her friend. In this way, she may be working to separate herself from self-defeating relational patterns she internalized from her family. Instead, she might relate to her friend in the way the therapist relates to her. Yet, she may express empathy her own way, which may be different from the therapist's style. She has been influenced, but she is not modeling the therapist. She has incorporated something of the therapist into herself, thereby expanding her approach to feelings and relationships.

Growing autonomy may lessen an adolescent's need for approval, freeing her from a potentially constraining need to please. But unresolved longing for parental approval and love may cause a patient to become preoccupied with her therapist's reactions, dwelling not only on signs of affection and acceptance but also perceived slights or criticism that may disproportionately influence how she feels about herself. Rather than internalizing the therapist's influence to build her own life, she may, perhaps insidiously, begin to allow her therapist's opinions and reactions to drive personal decisions. When motivated by the wish to please, a patient can look like she is more independent than she, in fact, is, particularly because she may be eager to take in therapeutic input and follow recommendations. Therapists can be seduced into thinking that the patient is developing autonomy because she seems motivated to implement changes they have discussed, when in reality she is just trying to secure the therapist's approval. A patient's willingness to selectively take in therapeutic influence is different from efforts that are motivated by a wish for approval, even if, in both cases, the patient is following therapist suggestions. Regardless of how well she appears to be doing in treatment, a patient who is governed by longings for approval may be trapped by emotional dependence on her therapist.

A Patient May Feel More Prepared to Leave Treatment When She Has Developed Attachments Outside of Therapy

In the process of connecting to a therapist, a young woman is establishing an attachment outside of her family. She is creating a caregiving relationship that can support her efforts to be more autonomous from parents. The treatment relationship can also be a step toward establishing more mutually supportive relationships outside of treatment, which provide opportunity to apply what she has learned in therapy. As she gradually builds a stable base of peer relationships, she may feel less need for her therapist. This development may signal increased readiness to think about leaving treatment. The effort to form other supportive relationships can, in fact, be part of the process of separating from a therapist, and resistance to establishing these connections may reflect a lack of readiness to let go.

Group therapy can help a young woman transition from attachment to a therapist to mutually supportive, peer relationships. A group provides ready-made access to relationships, relieving a patient of the possibly daunting task of cultivating connections on her own before she is ready. Moreover, the group therapist might provide a secure base that helps a young woman open herself to more mutual relationships with group members. The feedback she gets in these therapeutically mediated interactions might help her to develop social skills and understand her interpersonal impact and the ways in which she falls into familiar, self-defeating roles.

This growing capacity for peer attachments may be part of what a patient will need to eventually leave her individual therapist. But if the transition to group is linked to "termination" of her individual therapy, it can interfere with a patient's ability to use her attachment to her therapist to deal with challenges posed by a group. Rather than replacing individual therapy, the addition of a group would complement and enhance the dyadic clinical work. Group experience makes possible more peer interaction than the patient might be able to generate if she is forced to draw exclusively from her social life. The patient's response to group also provides information about her approach to attachments outside of therapy as well as the nature of her attachment to the therapist—does she use her connection with her therapist to support or obstruct her connection with a group?

Melanie's therapist, Dr. H, referred her to one of my psychotherapy groups because he hoped that therapeutic peer contact would help her to become more genuine in social interactions. In the year that they had worked together, Melanie had developed an intense attachment to Dr. H. She relied on him to deal with self-doubt, anxiety, difficulty making decisions, and obsessive preoccupations (especially regarding others' perceptions of her).

Melanie was a twenty-seven-year-old graduate student with many friends and much dating experience, but her relationships tended to be superficial and offered little emotional support beyond the gratification she derived from feeling popular. She was so concerned about being liked by the people she admired that she was afraid to expose any sense of her emotional struggles or vulnerability.

Melanie agreed to enter group because she trusted Dr. H and probably also because she wanted to please him. But in group she remained distant and emotionally closed off. She said that she wanted to talk about problems only with Dr. H and her mother. She explained that no one else could understand her as well as they did. Melanie openly admitted that she felt no connection with me, and she did not even mention the possibility of getting support from group members. In fact, during this conversation, she did not even acknowledge the presence of anyone other than me.

Melanie revealed some vulnerability by acknowledging her dependence on Dr. H. But in the process, she devalued group members, who could reasonably feel unimportant or even irrelevant. Because she was forced to "share me" with others, I did not expect Melanie to make the kind of attachment to me that she had with Dr. H, so I was not surprised that she was reluctant to embrace a relationship with me. But she was even less receptive than I had expected. Her resistance to any meaningful relationship outside of Dr. H suggested that she might have been determined to maintain an exclusive attachment to him.

However, by telling us how she felt, Melanie was making some progress. The negative feedback she delivered was a striking departure for her—she was accustomed to telling people only what she thought they wanted to hear. So I did not challenge her. Instead, I said that her willingness to be honest could be the beginning of a connection, but I emphasized that I did not want to push for it. To the extent that she could attach to me, I hoped that it would help her to reach out more to other group members. But it was possible that Melanie was so straightforward with us because she did not care what we thought about her. She had a level of regard for her friends that she did not have for group members, and she valued her individual therapist in a way that she did not appear to value me.

I confronted Melanie's tendency to distance herself from group members. She felt criticized by this feedback. It was possible that her injury suggested that she did care what I thought of her, but I suspected that she simply could not tolerate any criticism. (She might have been so careful to avoid offending her friends because she knew that she could be devastated by their negative reactions.) Melanie took this conflict as evidence that I did not understand her and that she could trust only her individual therapist.

Not long after, she quit group therapy. It was possible that her decision to leave the group could represent a step toward asserting some autonomy in relation to Dr. H—she was probably risking his disapproval by dropping out so quickly. But I think it was more likely that she was just not ready yet to make therapeutic attachments beyond the security of her private, dyadic relationship with Dr. H.

It was possible that Melanie's attachment to Dr. H might eventually help her establish other, more genuine relationships, but it was also possible that she might be using the exclusive nature of their bond to avoid dependence and vulnerability with other people. Such dependence on a therapeutic relationship can be regressive or progressive depending, in part, on how it impacts a patient's ability to establish and sustain other relationships. At this point, the influence of Melanie's attachment to Dr. H on her ability to form other intimate connections was still uncertain.

By contrast, my work with Cheryl, a thirty-five-year-old single woman with minimal family supports, illustrates the way in which a therapeutic attachment can provide a base for building and sustaining other attachments. Because she worked independently as a writer, Cheryl also lacked colleagues and access to the supportive structure of an academic or business organization. Her treatment therefore provided an important source of support. Cheryl used our relationship to build a level of romantic commitment that might not otherwise have been possible for her. The type of continuing therapeutic dependence that Cheryl displayed could appear to be regressive but was really progressive and therapeutic. She was making effective use of ongoing therapeutic attachment to serve some of the refueling functions that were not available to her within her family.

It had been a struggle for Cheryl to establish a steady dating relationship. She was afraid to open up to people, in part due to her experience of feeling criticized and dismissed by her overbearing mother. Her father had died when she was four years old, and Cheryl's mother had turned to her older brother as the "man of the house" and her surrogate husband. Unable to recover from the loss, Cheryl's mother became depressed. Consequently, Cheryl lost her mother's attention, and her emotional needs came to be regarded as a burden. Cheryl's mother felt competitive with her—she envied her daughter's youthful beauty and ability to attract men. Perhaps because of this resentment, she was unwilling to entertain her daughter's perspective, and she would become angry if Cheryl challenged her in any way. She would discount Cheryl's opinions and ridicule her feelings and preferences.

Because of this experience, Cheryl had difficulties with trust, particularly in close relationships. She had been able to attach to a boyfriend, Jeff, who, unlike her mother, was usually willing to consider her needs and negotiate. But he was opinionated and distractible and could readily turn his attention from her, which she had trouble differentiating from her mother's lack of interest in her as a separate person. Cheryl could be deeply hurt by conflicts that Jeff regarded as mundane. Jeff had a track record of compromise, but nonetheless, Cheryl was afraid he would try to impose his will without considering her needs and feelings. Consequently, when they were in conflict, Cheryl would almost immediately begin to think of breaking up with Jeff. She felt the only power she had in the relationship was the power to leave him.

When talking with me, Cheryl would recognize that Jeff was really not much like her mother, but she would lose this insight when they were in conflict. She used the therapy to deal with the fears and painful memories of childhood interactions with her mother that were triggered by Jeff. Her attachment to me was perhaps even more important than any insights we made. In my role as therapist, I could focus on her needs and attune to her feelings in a way that she could not expect in a more reciprocal peer relationship. Jeff would impose his needs in a way that I, as a professional caregiver, would not. For this reason, Cheryl's need for our attachment actually grew as her relationship with Jeff became more intimate.

After she moved in with Jeff, I wanted to help Cheryl tolerate the stress and frustration of daily interaction with him. I admitted to Cheryl that I felt that I might be filling in for what Cheryl perceived as Jeff's inadequacies. But it seemed important for me to provide what she appeared to need in order to tolerate his limitations. Jeff's difficulty sustaining attention on Cheryl's needs hit directly on her area of greatest vulnerability—given her experience with her mother, she was easily hurt by any failure to attend to her. Cheryl was not using my empathic connection with her to replace intimacy with others but rather to manage the stress and injury inherent in efforts to build a romantic relationship. The therapy enabled her to hold on to a more balanced and realistic picture of Jeff and remain more resilient in the face of the inevitable frustrations and injuries she would experience with him.

Letting a Patient Take the Lead in Separating

To support autonomy, therapists might need to communicate that they are receptive to talking about ending treatment. But if they go a step further and suggest that they think that the patient might be ready to end, they risk undermining her comfort maintaining the continuing connection that she may need. When a therapist raises the issue of termination, the patient can feel rejected or overly dependent. Moreover, the therapist risks appropriating the patient's initiative, depriving her of the opportunity to feel responsible for the separation.

A young woman may hesitate to acknowledge gain or emerging readiness to end therapy for fear that her sense of progress will not be validated by the therapist. Alternatively, she may fear that once she opens the door (by raising the question of termination), her therapist will push her out. She may also be constrained by the concern that her desire to leave will hurt the therapist and, at the same time, that she will be hurt if the therapist lets her go too easily. The challenge for therapists is to be able to pick up on signs or signals that a patient might be thinking about ending treatment, while leaving the initiative and control in the hands of the patient.

For example, a young woman who has always tried to reschedule appointments when she has had to miss begins to cancel sessions without attempting to find an alternative time. Or, a patient who has always come to therapy with many issues to discuss begins to struggle to find things to talk about. In either case, the patient may be pulling back to avoid difficult issues. It is also possible that due to recent progress, she might have stalled because she needs help to redirect her therapeutic efforts. But the patient could also be communicating a lessening need for the therapy. She may have reached a point in the treatment where she is more able to deal with her feelings and relationships; minimize her vulnerability to crises, anxiety, or episodes of depression; anticipate therapeutic feedback; identify maladaptive patterns; and engage a broader network of social support. If therapists fail to recognize these changes, they can undermine movement toward autonomy, and therapy may begin to stagnate. If, on the other hand, therapists overreact and push toward termination, they may undermine the patient's need to pace the process.

Supporting Separation While Allowing for Continuing Attachment

If a young woman loses support from a caregiver—parent or therapist—as she tries to strike out on her own, she may feel less confident, less equipped to take potentially fruitful risks, and less able to recover from the inevitable disappointments and failures. Eager as she is to direct her life, she may be limited by the fact that she is operating without a net. Therapists who feel that their work is done when a patient leaves treatment are like parents who convert a daughter's bedroom into a den when she takes off for college. The daughter may never actually move back into her old room, but she benefits from knowing that she could if she wanted to. But if the caregiver is too eager to step in or does not establish a boundary that recognizes autonomy, a young woman may be unable to feel that she is really on her own and take pride in her in accomplishments.

By reducing the frequency of sessions in anticipation of ending therapy and remaining available afterward, therapists can provide a home base that serves as a reliable source of emotional refueling. In this effort, they may be able to compensate, to some extent, for a deficit in continuing support from parents who may have pulled back in response to their daughter's growing autonomy. To support independent development, therapists must be open to future contact without imposing expectation that the patient should necessarily take advantage of their continuing availability. A patient carries some responsibility to make appropriate use of the therapist's availability in accord with her needs. She must seek support or contact, as needed, and let go again when she has gotten enough.

A young woman who regards posttreatment contact as a sign of her failure may resist returning. The prospect of ending may feel more overwhelming, and the patient may have more difficulty after she does terminate, if she forecloses the possibility of follow-up or renewed therapeutic visits.

But some hesitance to renew therapeutic contact may be appropriate—a young woman needs to feel she is now on her own. The possibility of continued therapeutic contact can be used to deny the reality that this therapy experience is over. If a termination is regarded too much as a temporary break rather than an ending, or if therapy is allowed to peter out without addressing intent to end treatment, the patient may be deprived of opportunity to deal with the emotional impact of the separation. She may be able to gloss over the loss. A young woman may not think in terms of termination because she is not yet prepared to deal with the loss. It is also possible, however, that she may simply not regard her decision to stop sessions as an ending. Adolescents and young adults may instinctively think in terms of refueling and, as Eichler described in his work with college students, they may naturally move in and out of therapy. While using the therapeutic relationship as a foundation, patients might separate incrementally.

Therapists need to exercise restraint in their approach to posttreatment contact. If they are eager to jump back into their former role, they may re-create familiar interaction, causing a young woman to fall back into the role of "patient" when she had wanted to relate from a different position. She may come in to celebrate a milestone in her life, but if the therapist homes in on feelings of anxiety, for example, instead of her sense of accomplishment, she may come to believe that she needs more help than perhaps she had thought. She may, for example, begin to crave the reassurance that the therapist provided in the past. If therapists instead attend to and appreciate new dimensions of the patient's capacities, they can introduce increased mutuality into the treatment relationship that recognizes and supports her autonomy.

Embracing the Risks
Inherent in Separation

I return now to my ambivalence regarding Belle's planned termination from a partial hospital program. A few weeks after she raised her intent to end, I learned that Belle had started a steady dating relationship. It was a big departure for her to become intimately involved with anyone. Perhaps I should have been more encouraged and enthusiastic than I was. But I felt concerned about her choice of partners. Sam did not seem trustworthy. I learned that when they began having sex, he did not tell Belle that he had herpes, so she could not make an informed decision about how she might want to deal with it. Nor did he try to protect her by using a condom. Consequently, Belle contracted the virus. I was concerned about Belle in this relationship, but also about whether her decision to become seriously involved with Sam might signal that she was not ready to leave the program.

I was not sure what to make of the fact that Belle did not seem angry about contracting herpes from Sam. Her response (or lack thereof) might have suggested regression to her old destructive patterns, but now she was using a relationship to hurt herself. She might have been trying to find a way to get me to hold up her discharge because, after initiating her plan, she no longer felt ready to leave. Belle undoubtedly was still grappling with self-destructive inclinations. But I also think that given all the pain and injury she had become accustomed to in her gymnastics training, herpes might not have seemed like a big deal to her.

I did not let my concerns about these risks overshadow my awareness of Belle's progress. She was opening herself to another person. Moreover, it was possible that Sam might not have told Belle about his herpes because he feared rejection, not because he wanted to hurt her. This relationship probably represented a mixture of her familiar attraction to dangerous or destructive experience along with new experience, including some genuine intimacy. If I fixated on the potential dangers and failed to recognize progressive aspects of her behavior, I could push Belle back toward more regressive choices. With Sam, she might be beginning to build a relationship that not only reflected therapeutic gain but also might provide some of support the she would need after she left the program. It would be important for Belle to become more involved with peer relationships, and I wanted to support any attachment she might make.

Therapists facing termination struggle with some of the fears and ambivalence that a parent might experience in launching their daughter. There is always some question whether a young woman will sustain therapeutic gains and manage her problems after she leaves therapy, and there is an element of uncertainty and risk associated with autonomy, particularly for someone with a history of self-destructive behavior.

But my struggle with Belle's proposed termination was heightened by longstanding dynamics in our relationship. Throughout Belle's treatment, I had consistently been in the role of identifying and confronting her possible secret destructive behavior or disguised destructive intent. I would learn of vomiting and laxative abuse, for example, only if I noticed and asked about swelling in her face. I was primed by Belle to be suspicious, to wonder what destructive behavior she might be hiding. This "cat-and-mouse" interaction was part of our relationship, and it was unlikely that we would entirely work our way out of the pattern, which had been so central to our attachment.

Belle's passivity in the face of potential danger would make me want to "drag" information out of her and try to frighten her into protective action. I sometimes felt heavy-handed and intrusive in our interactions. She was able to provoke an aggressive element in our relationship that was familiar and probably exciting to her. My role was to suspect her motives, to chase her down, and to press her to admit to self-destructive behavior or intent. This pattern probably held some masochistic gratification for Belle, but it also expressed both my frustrated and protective feelings for her. She both resisted and internalized my protective efforts. I think that overall our struggle helped her to begin taking better care of herself.

After I learned about her relationship with Sam, I confronted Belle about her failure to protect herself when they had sexual relations. In that interaction, Belle had said nothing to reassure me or to show that she even registered the risk, which further provoked my concern. Several weeks later, Belle told me that she had been hurt by my disapproval. She needed me to support this relationship despite its potential risks, and appreciate her progress. I told her that I did not disapprove of the relationship and that, in fact, I knew little about Sam. My worries came largely from what she had told me—she might feel differently about risks than I did, but she had recognized them herself. I further pointed out that she had shared little of what she liked about Sam, then she criticized me for not accepting him. When she thought about this, she laughed, recognizing the position in which she had put me. This was a moment of genuine, intimate connection. Through her willingness to laugh, Belle acknowledged that she played a role in our cat-and-mouse pattern of interaction.

As far as I could tell, Belle was beginning to let go of her overtly self-destructive behaviors. She was not as self-protective as I would have hoped, but she was also less destructive than she had been, and her choice of Sam was probably infused with some recklessness, but it seemed preponderantly progressive. Our pattern of relating persisted—her continued reticence helped to perpetuate a polarization in which I was the vigilant, suspicious one, on guard for self-imposed danger, and she placidly embraced worrisome developments in her life. But she was no longer hurting herself and our "cat-and-mouse" pattern of interaction might have represented a healthier, more related manner of containing her destructive impulses. Belle would oppose my therapeutic influence, resist my efforts to pull for more disclosure, and dispute my concerns. But she also seemed attached to this struggle. Although our conflict could defend against intimacy, it also provided an intense emotional connection. When she left the program, I would miss her.

I recognized that Belle was struggling with conflicting regressive and progressive motives, as she would likely continue to do. She now had internalized some self-protective interest that allowed her to struggle rather than simply run headlong toward self-deprivation and injury. For this reason, I could very genuinely share with Belle my appreciation of the growth in her personal life. That I could not stop her from acting self-destructively and that I could not even know, with any certainty, whether her choices were destructive drove home the reality of Belle's autonomy and her separateness even within the context of our attachment.

Accepting the Limitations
of What Therapy Can Provide

To commit to treatment, to stay engaged through frustrations and challenges, and to leave feeling satisfied, a young woman must be able to value her therapist despite his or her inevitable clinical and personal shortcomings. "The patient who finds a way to appreciate and cultivate the value of the analytic relationship, despite its glaring limitations, may well create a model for his or her being able to embrace and make the most of other relationships as well" (Hoffman, 1998, p. 12).

If she is to take advantage of potential for new experience in relationships, a young woman must mourn the loss of what she did not get from parents in childhood. By looking to parents to compensate for their past failures, she may become trapped by her anger and unfulfilled longings. Belated parental caregiving efforts may be taken as an expression of guilt or a wish to silence a daughter's anger and disappointment, and consequently they might feel less genuine and fulfilling. Because these efforts were not made when they were most needed, they may seem "too little, too late." Yet, by dismissing their value altogether, a daughter may lose an opportunity to create some experience of closeness with parents in adulthood, wherein mutuality might be expressed by her willingness to accept their past and current limitations. Similarly, if she looks to peers to provide the unconditional love that she did not get from parents, she may become disillusioned with these relationships as well, and unable to take in and build upon the love and care that *is* available to her. She may repeat the frustration and deprivation from her childhood as she continues to seek what has eluded her rather than allowing herself to appreciate what is attainable.

By mourning this loss, however, a patient can create a different kind of hope—the hope that her needs can be met well enough in relationships that are available. To realize this possibility, she must recognize that getting less than what she wants is different from getting nothing. Like the effort to launch from family, termination challenges a young woman to come to terms with what a caregiver has failed to provide, and also to recognize and hold onto what has been of value that she might carry forward into other relationships. She will hopefully feel readier to move from a caregiving attachment to peer relationships, where her emotional needs can be met through more mutual and shared efforts to nurture each other.

References

Abelin, E. (1971). The role of the father in the separation–individuation process. In J. B. McDevitt & C. F. Settlage (Eds.), *Separation–Individuation: Essays in Honor of Margaret S. Mahler* (pp. 229–253). New York: International University Press.

Ainsworth, M. (1963). The development of infant–mother interaction among the Ganda. In B. M. Foss (Ed.), *Determinants of infant behavior* (Vol. 2, pp. 67–112). New York: Wiley.

Allen, J. P., & Land, D. (1999). Attachment in adolescence. In J. Cassidy & P. R. Shaver (Eds.), *Handbook of attachment: Theory, research, and clinical applications* (pp. 319–335). New York: Guilford Press.

Balint, M. (1968). *The basic fault: Therapeutic aspects of regression*. Evanston, IL: Northwestern University Press.

Benjamin, J. (1988). *The bonds of love: Psychoanalysis, feminism, and the problem of domination*. New York: Pantheon Books.

Blos, P. (1962). *On Adolescence: A psychoanalytic interpretation*. New York: Free Press.

Blos, P. (1968). Character formation in adolescence. *Psychoanalytic Study of the Child, 23,* 245–264.

Bowlby, J. (1988). *A secure base: Clinical applications of attachment theory.* New York: Brunner-Routledge.

Cassidy J., & Berlin, L. F. (1994). The insecure/ambivalent pattern of attachment: Theory and research. *Child Development, 65,* 971–991.

Chodorow, N. J. (1978). *The reproduction of mothering: Psychoanalysis and the sociology of gender.* Berkeley: University of California Press.

Chodorow, N. J. (1998). Feminism and difference: Gender, relation, and difference in psychoanalytic perspective. In B. M. Clinchy & J. K. Norem (Eds.), *The gender and psychology reader* (pp. 347–405). New York: New York University Press. (Originally published in 1979).

Cooper, S. H., & Levit, D. (2005). Old and new objects in Fairbairnian and American relational theory. In L. Aron & A. Harris (Eds.), *Relational psychoanalysis: Vol. 2. Innovation and expansion* (pp. 51–74). Hillsdale, NJ: Analytic Press.

Davies, J. M., & Frawley, M. G. (1994). *Treating the adult survivors of childhood sexual abuse.* New York: Basic Books.

Davies, J. M., & Frawley, M. G. (1999). Dissociative processes and transference–countertransference paradigms in the psychoanalytically oriented treatment of adult survivors of childhood sexual abuse. In S. A. Mitchell & L. Aron (Eds.), *Relational psychoanalysis: The emergence of a tradition* (pp. 269–304). Hillsdale, NJ: Analytic Press. (Originally published in 1991).

Doctors, S. R. (2000). Attachment–individuation: I. Clinical notes toward a reconsideration of "adolescent turmoil." *Adolescent Psychiatry, 25,* 3–16.

Ehrenberg, D. B. (1992). *The intimate edge: Extending the reach of psychoanalytic interaction.* New York: Norton.

Eichler, R. J. (2006). Developmental considerations. In P. A. Grayson & P. W. Meilman (Eds.), *College mental health practice* (pp. 21–42). New York: Routledge.

Freud, A. (1975). Adolescence. In A. H. Esman (Ed.), *The psychology of adolescence* (pp. 122–140). New York: International Universities Press. (Original work published 1958).

Gilligan, C. (1993). *In a different voice: Psychological theory and women's development.* Cambridge, MA: Harvard University Press. (Originally published in 1982).

Hoffman, I. Z. (1998). *Ritual and Spontaneity in the psychoanalytic process: A dialectical-constructivist view.* Hillsdale, NJ: Analytic Press.

Hoffman, I. Z. (2006). Forging difference out of similarity: The multiplicity of corrective experience. *Psychoanalytic Quarterly, 75*(3), 715–751.

Holmes, J. (1996). *Attachment, intimacy, autonomy: Using attachment theory in adult psychotherapy.* Northvale, NJ: Aronson.

Lyons-Ruth, K. (1991). Rapprochement and approchement: Mahler's theory reconsidered from the vantage point of recent research on early attachment relationships. *Psychoanalytic Psychology, 8*(1), 1–23.

Mahler, M. S. (1979). *Separation–individuation: The selected papers of Margaret S. Mahler* (Vol. II). Northvale, NJ: Aronson.

Mahler, M. S., Pine, F., & Bergman, A. (1975). *The psychological birth of the human infant: Symbiosis and Individuation.* New York: Basic Books.

Marohn, R. (1998). A reexamination of Peter Blos's concept of prolonged adolescence. *Adolescent Psychiatry, 23,* 3–20.

McLaughlin, J. T. (1995). Resistance. In B. E. Moore & B. D. Fine (Eds.), *Psychoanalysis: The major concepts* (pp. 95–109). New Haven, CT: Yale University Press.

McWilliams, N. (2004). *Psychoanalytic psychotherapy: A practitioner's guide.* New York: Guilford Press.

Mitchell, S. A. (1988). *Relational concepts in psychoanalysis: An integration.* Cambridge, MA: Harvard University Press.

Mitchell, S. A. (1993). *Hope and dread in psychoanalysis.* New York: Basic Books.

Mitchell, S. A. (1997). *Influence and autonomy in psychoanalysis.* Hillsdale, NJ: Analytic Press.

Mitchell, S. A., & Black, M. J. (1995). *Freud and beyond: A history of modern psychoanalytic thought.* New York: Basic Books.

Perl, E. (1997a). Breaking up or breaking away: The struggle around autonomy and individuation among adolescent daughters of divorce. *Adolescent Psychiatry, 21,* 83–99.

Perl, E. (1997b). The treatment team in conflict: The wishes for and risks of consensus. *Psychiatry: Interpersonal and Biological Processes. 60*(2), 182–195.

Perl, E. (1998). Snatching defeat from the jaws of success: Self-destructive behavior as an expression of autonomy in young women. *Adolescent Psychiatry, 23,* 143–170.

Ryan, R. M., & Lynch, J. H. (1989). Emotional autonomy versus detachment: Revisiting the vicissitudes of adolescence and young adulthood. *Child Development, 60,* 340–356.

Safran, J. D., & Muran, J. C. (2000). *Negotiating the therapeutic alliance: A relational treatment guide.* New York: Guilford Press.

Slade, A.(1999). Attachment theory and research: Implications for the theory and practice of individual psychotherapy with adults. In J. Cassidy & P. R. Shaver (Eds.), *Handbook of attachment: Theory, research, and clinical applications* (pp. 575–594). New York: Guilford Press.

Slochower, J. (2005) Holding: Something old and something new. In L. Aron & A. Harris (Eds.), *Relational psychoanalysis, Vol. 2: Innovation and expansion* (pp. 29–49). Hillsdale, NJ: Analytic Press. (Original work published 1996).

Winnicott, D. (1949). Hate in the countertransference. *International Journal of Psychoanalysis, 30,* 69–74.

Index